Dear God, Bless This Mess

What Christians Should Know About Food, Health & Healing

Amanda Roberson, ND, M.Ed.

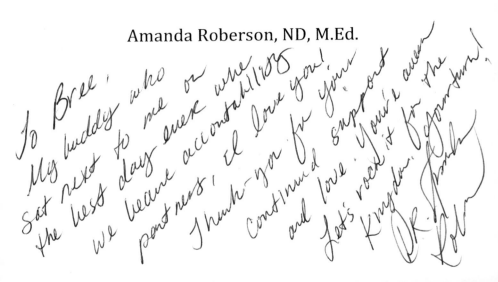

To Bree,
My buddy who sat next to me on the best day ever when we became accountability partners, I love you! Thank you for your continued support and love. You're awesome! Let's rock it for the Kingdom!
Dr. Amanda Rob

Editing by: Exclamation Publishing
Cover by: Clarity Consulting & Design

The information in this book represents the viewpoint and experiences of the author. It is not intended to replace or supersede medical advice from your physician. For this reason, the author/publisher is not responsible or liable for any injury or loss incurred for any individuals who use the information presented in the text to self-treat. Readers must seek recommendations from and be supervised by a qualified health professional.

Contents

Dedication

This book is dedicated to my Lord and Savior Jesus Christ. Thank you for loving me and giving Yourself for me to have victory. You are amazing, and I honor You with my life! Thank you for inspiring me to push through the "business" of life to complete the book for the benefit of others. I would also like to thank my family and friends in Atlanta as well as my extended family at Faith Christian Center in Phoenix for their continued support regarding this project.

Introduction

It's time to be completely transparent. The moment has arrived. We must give account and "fess up" about our current eating habits. We need to admit to God and ourselves what we are *really* doing.

Does the following prayer sound somewhat familiar? "Dear Lord, please bless the food that I'm about to receive. Help it to nourish and strengthen my body in Jesus' name I pray. Amen." If it sounds relatively familiar or if the intention of the prayer sounds similar to what you typically say for grace before eating, you're not alone. Daily, Christians give thanks and ask God to bless the food they eat. However, it would be interesting to note the nutritional content more closely in the food being prayed over and its biochemical capacity to actually "nourish and strengthen" the consumer. Considering most food available in the United States, it's likely that the foods would not provide substantial nourishment. In contrast, there would likely be an excess of unhealthy fats coupled with copious amounts of sugar and salt. Sadly, this is typical of the Standard American Diet (SAD), which is appropriately abbreviated. With this in mind, take a moment to consider the following question: How do you think God feels about us praying for His blessing over food that we know is not *really* good for us?

God, abundant with grace and mercy, has designed our bodies masterfully. Yet, He also entrusts us to care for these vessels of clay so His Spirit will have somewhere to reside so He can operate on Earth. Are you doing your part in this arrangement or are you essentially tempting the Lord regarding your health by doing something you know will ultimately yield no benefits? First Corinthians 10:23 (AMP) states that "all things are legitimate [permissible—and we are free to do anything we please], but not all things are helpful (expedient, profitable, and wholesome). All things are legitimate, but not all things are constructive [to character] *and* edifying [to spiritual life]." Therefore, since you have committed your life to God, it's time to learn how to proactively make necessary changes to your diet to take better care of your temple. As an added bonus, you will be healthy and have lots of energy to do the things God wants you to do.

Right now, you might be thinking, "Easier said than done, Dr. Amanda." I understand and know that becoming healthy can seem overwhelming! As medical knowledge has increased, a plethora of information now exists. With so much to read and learn, how do you know what's *really* good for you and what is just hype? For this reason, this book is intended for Christians who want abundant, healthy lives as God intends, but are not confident about how to change their daily habits, because of conflicting information, limited access, tradition, or even lack of motivation to change.

Proverbs 18:21 states that "death and life are in the power of the tongue, and they who indulge in it shall eat the fruit of it [for death or life]." Although this verse has been interpreted in other biblical translations to relate to spoken words, there are also valid reasons to consider that it may also relate to what one eats. This book will provide an overview about how the food we eat actually does impact our health—both short and long-term. Research has demonstrated that what we eat can have a negative or positive effect on our health. Additionally, there is also a cumulative effect based on what you eat long-term. Depending on your age, your choices may have an even greater influence on your health. Also, if you have children or want to in the future, your choices can effect them and future generations to come.

As a naturopathic physician, one guiding principle I use to care for patients is prevention. By teaching about viable options and alternatives that improve health, many of the most common chronic diseases in the United States could be completely thwarted. Remember you can bring God glory and honor in your life by making an intentional effort to take better care of the body God entrusted to you. I'm delighted to teach you how!

A Prayer for You

Dear God,

Please bless everyone who reads this book! Help them to recognize the importance of the decisions they make about food. Grant them wisdom regarding how to feasibly make better choices and to make lifestyle transitions as necessary with ease. Help them to learn and recall the information presented in this book and as a result, eagerly take initiative to better care for their bodies. God, thank You for healing any illness or disease that concerns them, and guiding them toward health and healing, which You have already preordained for Your children. Amen.

~

While reading this book, in an effort to improve your results, say the confessions that follow aloud on a regular basis. By speaking these scripture-based confessions, you will use your words as a weapon against the enemy. The more you recite them, the easier it will be for you to have faith, and you will see results manifested in your life because God's Word works!

Confessions For You

My life is valuable, important and significant so I glorify God with my body. My body is the temple of the Holy Spirit. (1 Corinthians 6:19-20)

God keeps me in perfect peace about my health because my mind is stayed on Him. (Isaiah 26:3)

Jesus was pierced for my transgressions, He was crushed for my iniquities; the punishment that brings me peace was on Him, and by His wounds I am healed. (Isaiah 53:5)

Although everything is permissible for me, I know that all things are not beneficial, and the Holy Spirit helps me distinguish the difference. (1 Corinthians 10:23)

My body prefers healthy foods that nourish and strengthen it so it functions properly. I do not crave unhealthy processed foods. As a result, my mind is alert, and I have more energy to be about my Father's business. (Luke 2:49)

Exercising regularly is good for me. I enjoy training my body physically, and I am growing stronger in spirit as well. (1 Corinthians 9:24-27)

Holy Spirit I give You liberty to guide my decisions about how to care for the body God entrusted to me. The same power that raised Jesus from the dead is at work in me helping me to be healthy and live victoriously! (Ephesians 1:19-20)

Chapter One: New Beginnings

The Purpose of Food

One of my sisters has a Havanese dog named Benny. Recently, she told me something funny about her beloved dog. She said, "He lives to eat!" The joy of his life is eating, particularly the foods that people eat. Every time someone goes into the kitchen, he's acutely aware and strategically positions himself in a manner that enables him to direct those irresistible big, brown eyes toward the person who can help him enjoy life ... at least for the few seconds he gobbles up the treat tossed in his direction.

So now it's time for transparency again. Are we like Benny—strategizing and planning our lives around the pleasure of food? As humans made in the image of God, shouldn't we expect a bit more from ourselves? Yes, eating can be enjoyable, and we must eat to survive long-term. However, which part of us usually makes the decision regarding the quality or quantity of food we eat? Is it the instinctive, canine part of our flesh that craves food, which is the most basic form of satisfaction? Or is it our intellect that decides the food we eat has to be desirable? Many of us probably relate to Benny and make decisions about food simply based on cravings. Now, some of you may be wondering, "Should we *really* default the decisions we make regarding what to eat to our spirits?" Perhaps, we should since our spirits operate in sync with the Holy Spirit, Who knows all things.

If this sounds too spiritual, we have to remember that God is the Creator of food. Of course He wants us to enjoy it! But God's primary intention was for food to be a source of nourishment. In Genesis 1:29, God tells Adam, "See, I have given you every plant yielding seed that is on the face of all the land and every tree with seed in its fruit; you shall have them for food." Later in Genesis 9:3, God tells Noah, "Every moving thing that lives shall be food for you; and as I gave you the green vegetables *and* plants, I give you everything." Based on these passages, it is apparent that God wanted us to eat vegetables, fruits, and moving things, which likely meant animals. Considering God's divine design of our bodies, He knew we would need nourishment in some form for energy production and provided clear options for us. These specific sources of fuel for the body were meant and intended to provide nutrients like vitamins, minerals, and healthy fats along with reasonable proportions of carbohydrates. However, because food has drastically changed since Adam and Noah were given instructions about what to eat, it seems reasonable for us as Christians to become more attentive and knowledgeable regarding what we choose to eat.

The First Temptation

Let's take a moment to venture back to the beginning of time. Here's a biblical scholar quiz question. True or False: The first sin committed on the Earth had something to do with eating something? That's right! The answer is true. Isn't that interesting? The very first sin committed by Adam and Eve was that they ate the forbidden fruit of the tree of the knowledge of good and evil. Another interesting point is that Eve had not been created at the time God gave the original instruction. Only Adam existed. Apparently, Adam warned Eve not to eat of the tree. Unfortunately, it seems either Adam didn't provide clear instructions or Eve didn't understand the seriousness of the matter. When God tells us to avoid doing something, it's always for our own protection. However, Eve chose to abide in the flesh and satisfy her lustful desire for the forbidden fruit.

Now, let's take the same scenario but change the setting to your dinner table. Do *you* recognize the seriousness of the food you eat or do you have on sporty, rose-colored glasses? Sometimes temptation occurs because the flesh simply goes after what it wants by default. Perhaps you've been desensitized to God's input concerning your food choices or maybe you haven't asked Him for input yet. On other occasions, the enemy may present tantalizing opportunities for you to partake of the beloved food you crave, because he knows the long-term consequences of your preferred food choices—a deceptively slow, early death.

Do you remember when Jesus was being tempted by the devil to cast Himself off the pinnacle of the temple? His response to the enemy was, "You shall not tempt, test thoroughly, or try exceedingly the Lord your God."[1] The devil was essentially trying to get Jesus to commit suicide to ruin and destroy God's will from taking place. In a similar manner, when we are tempted to consistently eat things that are not beneficial for our health, this could also be perceived as a form of suicide, albeit a slow form of self-sabotage that does not conspicuously ascribe responsibility to the individual.

God has given us free will to choose. We decide whether or not we will follow His leading in everything—our careers, marriages, friendships, purchases, trips, business opportunities, actions, thoughts, and even what we choose to eat daily. God's Word says "I [the Lord] will instruct you and teach you in the way you should go; I will counsel you with My eye upon you. Be not like the horse or the mule, which lack understanding, which must have their mouths held firm with bit and bridle, or else they will not come with you."[2] Apparently, God's intention is not to force us to do His will. Instead, He is searching our hearts seeking out willing vessels that will yield to Him—completely. This is where He can really use us for His glory. How much of your every day life is *really* yielded to the Holy Spirit? Let's aim for 100 percent!

Here's a challenge: Yield. Allow the Holy Spirit to confirm or even refute your food choices and follow His leading. Eat to live! You might be surprised how your diet changes. You'll be even more surprised by how great you can feel regardless of your age!

Chapter Two: Law & Prayer

<u>The Law</u>

When God designed everything, He created it all with physical, chemical, and biological organization and patterns. For example, the law of gravity, which keeps things from floating away, is operating right now helping you hold the book or electronic device in your hand while you read in the comfortable location you've chosen. Other basic laws of physics are currently at work regardless of your awareness of them. Try to move a small object near you. See! An object at rest will remain at rest unless an outside force acts upon it. Based on the way chemistry works, most people know mixing baking soda and vinegar will produce lots of bubbles and burning wood or coal produces gas and heat. Lastly, biological laws persist as well. For example, in autumn each year, deciduous trees automatically cease production of chlorophyll, which originally makes the leaves green when they appear in the spring. As a result, other pigments that were in the leaves when they initially emerged can be seen like carotenoids (yellow and orange) and anthocyanins (red).[3] In the same way that other aspects of creation abide by these God-ordained laws, our bodies function based on laws and principles too. If these laws are broken, disregarded, or ignored, there will *certainly* be consequences.

Did you happen to watch the film documentary *Supersize Me* by Morgan Spurlock? This documentary illustrated how regular consumption of fast food and a lack of physical activity is not ideal for health for a myriad of reasons. In the same way, similar results would be likely if an inactive person consistently ate packaged foods purchased from the local grocery store. Packaged foods typically contain unhealthy forms of fats and proteins along with excessive carbohydrates, sugar, and salt. In general, they are nutritionally deficient, which is why fortification and enrichment are necessary.

Now, suppose a person ate what is considered a relatively "healthy" diet based on the food typically available in America. In addition to eating some quickly prepared homemade meals, let's suppose they ate out regularly at restaurants and managed to workout a couple of times each week. What consequences do you think this person might experience? Finally, contrast this example with the person who intentionally becomes informed about how diet and lifestyle impact health, seeks out resources and strategies from competently trained professionals, and then implements significant positive changes in their regimen. The latter person will ultimately benefit from basic laws that govern health both as a result of their intention and execution through a disciplined lifestyle. Health doesn't happen coincidentally, but is the summation of daily lifestyle choices.

The Truth of the Matter

Just as jumping off of bridges renders consequences based on the laws of physics, in the same way, eating lots of unhealthy foods that increase inflammation and bad cholesterol in the body will lead to negative consequences as well. Unfortunately, the consequences of poor health choices are not noticed as quickly. They are deceptive processes. Having a chronic disease *is* due to choices made over a long period of time so the repercussions are not as apparent when initial problems begin. As many of us get older, chronic disease becomes inevitable based on sedentary lifestyles and cumulative years of unhealthy food choices.

Based on preliminary 2011 data available from the Centers for Disease Control and Prevention (CDC), the following are the 10 leading causes of death in America[4]:

1. Heart Disease
2. Cancer
3. Chronic Lower Respiratory Disease
4. Cerebrovascular Disease
5. Accidents
6. Alzheimer's Disease
7. Diabetes Mellitus
8. Influenza & Pneumonia
9. Kidney Disease
10. Suicide

Notably, many of the leading causes of death can be related to lifestyle and dietary choices. Extensive research supports the idea that implementing a consistent and relatively rigorous exercise regimen coupled with a healthy diet can prevent many of these diseases. Yet, although we know this is truth, implementation and consistency seems to be a huge obstacle for many people.

Based on statistics, the chemical and biological laws that govern our health seem to be disregarded and ignored based on the evident, pervasive health crisis in America. While diagnoses of chronic diseases continue to rise, there is an elusive culprit whose intention has always been to kill, steal, and destroy.[5] As believers, our adversary the devil is actively seeking whom he may devour.[6] The enemy is using stealthy strategies to attempt to extinguish the body of Christ without our awareness of it. Unfortunately, many Christians have grown oblivious and insensitive to the fact that what they eat *is* a spiritual battle and succumb to being distracted by the "cares of the world."[7] This may be why we see such little distinction between the body of Christ and others who do not believe. We should be producing fruit, yet we've been numbed by our excessive ways of eating and living. It's time to choose health! It's time to fight! We *can* do all things through Christ Who strengthens us.[8]

Identity and Purpose

As "aliens, strangers and exiles in the world," we should intentionally endeavor to remain focused on our purpose and avoid distractions that "wage war against the soul." [9]

> "Do not conform to the pattern of this world, but be transformed by the renewing of your mind. Then you will be able to test and approve what God's will is—His good, pleasing and perfect will."[10]

By remaining focused on our purpose, God is able to achieve His will. Unfortunately, if our focus is on hot, fresh glazed donuts, God's will being done on earth won't be expedient. Just imagine if Jesus had come during this day and age. The disciples, having succumbed to desires of their flesh as most of us do, would likely have elevated cholesterol, high blood sugar, and clogging arteries. Over time they would start to experience shortness of breath on exertion, which would make it extremely difficult to keep up with Jesus since He enjoyed walking and interacting with people. Perhaps only one or two of the disciples would be fit enough to go into all the world recruiting more disciples for God's kingdom. It really would be a mess!

For this reason, remember what 1 John 2:15-16 says regarding the matter: "Love not the world, neither the things that are in the world. If any man love the world, the love of the Father is not in him."[11] Ultimately, we must recognize that love is commitment. Since we can't serve two masters, we must choose whom we will serve or commit our lives to—God or things of this world (including food).[12, 13]

Fight Fair with Prayer

Based on the following, decide if each statement is true or false:

___ God grants us everything we pray for.

___ God wants us to be sick so when we pray He can heal us.

___ Praying over food, regardless of what it is, makes it acceptable to eat without consequence.

Hopefully, it was simple to notice that all of the statements above are false. Prayer is most effective when it is God's will. Thus, as Christians, we shouldn't expect that because we have a direct connection to God Who created the universe that He will be at our beckoning call when we present our prayer requests. This isn't how prayer works. When the disciples asked Jesus to teach them how to pray, Jesus' response was the Lord's Prayer in Matthew 6:9-13. It was an eloquent demonstration of reverence, submission, and dependence on God. In the same way, when we pray, the purpose should be to show God that we honor Him. It also serves as a reminder that we are totally dependent on Him for everything. In addition, prayer is a conversation between God and you. Take time during prayer to listen to what He wants since our omniscient Father knows everything. Humble hearts please God. When we commit our lives to Him, He will direct our paths as well as our prayers.

As the body of Christ, we are on God's team, and He clearly wants the best for us. However, we must recognize that nothing can happen on the earth (i.e. in the physical realm) until we either pray for it to occur or take action regarding what the Holy Spirit is leading us to do. This is how it has been since the beginning, and we must yield ourselves to work with God so His kingdom can come and His will can be done.

God's will is for us to be healthy, not sick. Since it is not God's will for us to be sick, we must abide in faith regarding this matter and mix our faith with corresponding action. There are numerous ways to take care of our bodies that significantly decrease the probability of sickness from being established in our bodies. These actions may include adopting lifelong habits like eating healthy foods, drinking sufficient water, and exercising regularly. We also can renew our minds daily by speaking the Word of God over ourselves with confessions and prayers. When we say God's Word aloud in faith, this action activates the power of the Word of God. Since God's Word will not return to Him void,[14] we are empowered to see results manifested by saying His Word with boldness and authority. This is a more effective way to pray.

Finally, another means of fighting fair with prayer is by praying in your heavenly language. The Bible says when we have the Holy Spirit living in us, there is evidence of His presence when we pray in unknown tongues.[15,16] What's really awesome about this type of prayer is that the devil doesn't know what you're praying so he can't attempt to sabotage the plan. In addition, you probably don't know what you're praying either, (unless you ask the Holy Spirit for the interpretation) so your personal ambitions and pursuits can't alter God's plans. When you pray in tongues, also known as praying in the Spirit, you pray God's perfect will. So, it's imperative that the body of Christ "pray at all times (on every occasion, in every season) in the Spirit with all [manner of] prayer and entreaty."[17] After all, prayer is a fundamental and empowering tactic that we can use to successfully "extinguish *all* of the flaming arrows of the evil one."[18] We must use every weapon and strategy provided for us to win. It's time to fight right!

~

Based on what is understood about the basic principles and laws that govern health, let's do our part to care for the temples God has loaned to us. Let's glorify God in our bodies. Let's use these vessels to do His work on the earth. Let's pray effectively in agreement with God's Word and one another, even when we bless our food, expecting positive changes to begin and continue taking place.

Chapter Three: You Really Are What You Eat

The You-Print: A Perfect Pattern

I will praise You, for I am fearfully *and* wonderfully made; Marvelous are Your works, and *that* my soul knows very well.[19]

Within the past century, the cellular blueprint used for the creation of all living things was discovered—deoxyribonucleic acid, more commonly called DNA. DNA is genetic material that's nestled within the cells of all the organisms God created. This wonderful compact, elegant structure holds the directions for the manifestation of our physical bodies. What's really fascinating about DNA is that it automatically performs its function daily.

An architectural blueprint of a house provides an appropriate analogy of DNA. Once the architect has worked with great tenacity to draw up plans for the home, materials are purchased to begin building the home. First, the foundation is set. Then the main frame of the home is erected. Next, floors, walls, and ceilings are installed with insulation where appropriate. Considerations are made for plumbing and electrical connections as well. Plastering, painting, and carpeting follow alongside installation of appliances. After adding decorative home furnishings, the house is ready to be a home!

In the same way, but on a smaller scale, sewing patterns are also a good metaphor for DNA. Quality material and suitable thread must be chosen to create a garment. In addition, special care must be taken when connecting each piece together to create one smooth cohesively structured clothing item. Using the pattern's guidelines, a garment can be produced that is meticulous and beautiful.

In each case, there's one underlying variable that can tremendously impact the outcome of the final product. Want to guess what it is? Yes, the *quality* of the materials chosen to build the house and construct the garment! If you've ever lived in a home that was built with quality materials and superb construction or if you've ever purchased high quality clothing, you *know* there's a distinct difference, especially after years or decades of use. Let's consider this concept as it relates to the body.

The TV show *Honey, We're Killing the Kids*, which previously aired on TLC, highlighted this concept based on the human body. During this reality TV program, a family with unhealthy dietary and lifestyle habits was shown how their current practices could impact the overall health and longevity of the children. What was particularly fascinating about the program was that the producers used computer technology to create images that projected what the kids would look like at age 40 if no changes were made. Truly, in this instance, a picture was worth a thousand words and likely triggered many unpleasant emotions in the parents as well.

DNA is your physical body's blueprint. You were constructed and "knitted together in your mother's womb."[20] Now, the blueprint simply provides instructions for maintenance. The construction material used to replenish and maintain your body is *entirely* based on what you eat and drink. Let's look at this more closely.

Biochemistry 101

The smallest unit of life is the cell. Your body is comprised of trillions of cells! Some of the cells replicate themselves and others die off according to information within the cell signaling if it is an appropriate reason or time to undergo *apoptosis*, which is essentially like "giving up the ghost" or deciding to die. At the same time, there are other cells, like many comprising the nervous system, that do not replicate, but continue to function as directed by DNA. Thus, there are numerous biochemical reactions taking place within each cell that are foundational for the optimal health of the whole organism.

Most of your body is water and a bunch of cells packed tightly together like sardines! There's also hair, which is primarily protein and fat.[21] Finally, there are areas where gas may exist either cooperatively or uncooperatively. Looking at the roles of each part of your body demonstrates its divine design.

Protein

Usually, when the word *protein* is mentioned, people typically think about meat like steak, chicken, or fish. Notably, there's so much more involved. Proteins take on a myriad of functions within the body and are all created from instructions that are saved within the DNA.

Here's a quick biological explanation about how DNA is

used to make protein. When a certain protein is needed, the DNA unwinds at a particular location so a complementary copy of DNA is formed. This copy is called the messenger RNA, or mRNA, which then moves out of the special cell compartment housing the DNA. The mRNA summons more support in protein production and an assembly assistant, ribosomal RNA (rRNA), attaches onto the mRNA. The rRNA essentially "reads" the mRNA's copied instructions in three unit segments that correspond to a specific amino acid. Then, the transfer assistant, tRNA, joins in the process by quickly bringing the necessary amino acid for the sequence to be linked together properly. After the amino acids have been linked together, the newly made protein may fold or bend based on positive and negative attractions of some of the amino acids. Finally, the protein is ready to serve its purpose! Some proteins that function in the body include the following[22]:

- Hemoglobin: Helps red blood cells carry oxygen throughout the body
- Insulin: Doubles as a hormone and assists cells in obtaining energy from food
- Collagen: Provides fibrous structure in the skin, blood vessels, and some parts of the eye
- Lactase: An enzyme that helps with digestion of lactose, which is a sugar found in milk products

Although elaborate, the point is important. There are 10 *essential* amino acids that must be consumed in the diet on a regular basis. This is why some foods are considered to be "complete" protein sources since they contain these required nutrients. Using other biochemical processes, if necessary, our bodies can make the other 10 amino acids necessary for protein synthesis. Thus, be mindful that the food you eat will be the source of about half of the proteins in your body and your DNA provides instructions for protein assembly.

Errors in protein synthesis can occur due to slight alterations in the DNA as in sickle cell anemia. Only one amino acid in the hemoglobin sequence is different. Errors may also occur due to excess production of a protein that becomes faulty over time as in type II diabetes. Oftentimes errors may go unnoticed for an extended time, but could potentially lead to deficits elsewhere. Thus, it's important to consume a diet that will support proper protein production.

Fat

The word *fat* may trigger varied emotions in some of us. Perhaps it triggers offense based on the shape of your body or your perception of it. Alternatively, your response may be a lustful desire to eat fatty foods, because they taste so good. Some people may even experience guilt because of a recent indulgence in a delightful, yet fatty treat. Regardless of your response, recognize that fat serves an important role in our bodies just like protein. In fact, fat comprises about 20 to 25 percent of the total weight of adults with normal weight.[23,24] In lieu of this, there's likely a reason we crave fatty foods since approximately 25 percent of our body is actually fat!

Fats vary in shape and size extensively based on the functions they serve within the body. For example, each cell in your body is surrounded by a membrane, which is an outer protective barrier comprised of a double layer of fats called *phospholipids*. Nestled within this fluid-like membrane are other fats like cholesterol and transport proteins that control what enters and exits the cells. When we consume quality types of fats, good things are allowed into the cells and wastes products are removed effectively. In contrast, when we eat unhealthy fats or disproportionate amounts of fats that are acceptable in moderation, the structure of the phospholipid bilayer is compromised so it cannot do its job efficiently. As a result, wastes may accumulate inside of our cells, and nutrients the cell needs cannot easily enter the cells.

Since the body is primarily comprised of water, which doesn't mix easily with oil, this poses a unique challenge for fat transport within the body. To facilitate this issue, oftentimes proteins are attached to fats so they can be transported throughout the body as needed. Also, some parts of fats (e.g. the head of a phospholipid) can interact with water more easily in comparison to the hydrophobic, or water repelling, fatty acid tail that does not mix well with water. Thus, the interaction phospholipids have with water encourages compartmentalization or packaging of fatty substances within spherical fat storage vesicles so they can move in and out of cells. In addition, freely circulating fats that easily interact with water are present throughout the body in various tissues to provide energy.[22] Some other functions of fats include helping the nervous system (including your brain) and immune system to function better. Fats are also used to make hormones like estrogen and testosterone, vitamins like vitamin D, and molecular messengers called prostaglandins.

Although the liver produces most of the cholesterol in our bodies, other fats that our bodies need to function are obtained from dietary sources.[25] Just as there are essential proteins we must obtain through our diets, there are also essential fats. Omega-3 and Omega-6 fatty acids help our bodies by decreasing inflammation, preventing platelets from sticking together and improving serum lipid levels that improve our health in a myriad of ways. Again, most of the good fats our bodies need must be obtained from dietary sources.

Unlike protein, which is produced based on information stored in the DNA, fat is synthesized through elaborate, strategic chemical reactions that involve mitochondria, little organ-like structures within cells that produce energy. The process is just as intricate as protein production, although there are no "blueprints," and these reactions are, for the most part, identical in everyone.

Notably, the body also converts any extra sugars into fat that is usually stored along the waistline of the body. Unfortunately, this fat does not offer health benefits other than being a potential energy source during a famine. This extra fat also contributes to increased production of stress hormone, or cortisol.

Minerals

Overall, minerals only make up a small percentage of our bodies. Although our bones contain high concentrations of calcium, most other minerals in our bodies are found in discrete quantities. Minerals have various functions "including the regulation of many enzymes by acting as cofactors, maintaining acid-base balance [and] osmotic pressure, facilitating transfer of essential compounds across membranes, maintaining proper nerve and muscle conduction and contraction, regulating growth of tissues, and making up critical components of structural tissue."[26] Specifically, magnesium assists in proper nerve function and is an extremely important cofactor for most B vitamins. Sodium and potassium work together to create energy for cells throughout the body by moving in opposite directions across cell membranes. This movement can also create an action potential along the surface of a cell to send a sensory signal like pain to the brain. Other minerals, such as zinc and selenium, are useful to improve immune system responses. Independently though, selenium assists significantly in detoxification processes, while zinc is particularly important for proper taste sensory function. Additionally, iron is found in heme, which is part of hemoglobin, a blood protein that carries oxygen. Finally, copper assists with cross-linking in connective tissue and is necessary for proper use of iron. Although generally overlooked in traditional medicine, many health concerns may be improved with proper mineral balance. Unfortunately, proper absorption of minerals tends to make maintaining optimal mineral levels challenging especially considering how food production has changed.

Carbohydrates

Although we are not technically comprised of carbohydrates, this is the preferred form of "fuel" our bodies use to function. With minimal effort, energy molecules called *adenosine triphosphate* or ATP can be produced to help other biochemical reactions occur and to warm our bodies simultaneously. Since this is a preferred quick fuel source, our livers store a small amount of carbohydrate in the form of glycogen to sustain us between meals if necessary. As noted previously, carbohydrates that have been broken down into simple sugars during digestion can be converted into fats and stored if too many carbs are consumed. This process will be addressed in more detail later.

****

NOTE: The proceeding sections of this chapter are quite technical and include lots of scientific terms. Please focus on simply having a better, general understanding about foods rather than getting bogged down by details. You are encouraged to seek out other supplemental resources to further expand your understanding as necessary.

Out With the New!

Our bodies need proteins, fats, minerals, and carbohydrates to function properly. The primary way to obtain these nutrients is through our food. However, in today's food market knowing what to eat is daunting. Most food currently available in the United States is produced on a large scale, processed to various extents, and packaged. For example, wheat is milled and whitened to become enriched flour for pastries; fruit is strained and the juice extracted is then concentrated, diluted, and sweetened with high fructose corn syrup; and chicken is separated mechanically, tainted with fillers and preservatives, seasoned with copious amounts of salt, and possibly laced with MSG.[27]

Another disturbing global concern is that there's mounting evidence that foods aren't as nutrient-dense as they were in the past.[28,29] Today, an apple does not contain the same amount of vitamins and other nutrients as apples from many years ago. In addition, pesticides are commonplace for large-scale food production and these chemicals (along with others from the environment) can eventually settle into our fluids and tissues, even in unborn babies![30] Another disconcerting issue is the relatively ubiquitous use of genetically altered products in many mainstream, common brands that contain ingredients such as corn, soy, or by-products from corn and soy.[31] Interestingly, many countries, excluding the United States, do not allow or permit foods with altered genes to be grown or sold to the public.[32] Perhaps this is due to uncertain health repercussions from such foods.

Due to these changes in our food, Christians must make an intentional effort to be well informed during the "information age" about the things we consume and how these things may affect our bodies. Remember "wisdom *is* the principal thing; *Therefore* get wisdom, and in all your getting, get understanding."[33] The remainder of this chapter will provide information about some of the ingredients in processed and packaged foods. Unfortunately, our new ways of cultivating, manufacturing, and processing food may be compromising our health based on the way our bodies were originally designed to function.

Fortunately, some positive changes are beginning to take place based on new government regulations. However, many more changes are necessary to have a significant positive impact on the overall health of Americans.

Trans-Fat

More than likely, you've heard of *trans-fat* and know that it is unhealthy for you. However, what you may not know is that prior to a recent government ruling in the summer of 2012 to ban trans-fat, the FDA allowed manufacturers to include trans-fat in their products as long as the total amount for each serving was no more than 0.5 grams. The government permitted companies to deceive consumers and claim that a product contained "0 grams of trans-fat" as long as each serving contained less than 0.5 grams of it. Deluded by this misleading allowance, many Americans probably consumed trans-fat in these products without knowing.

Well-informed consumers may not have been deceived so easily though. By reading ingredient labels, the savvy shopper would note some of the aliases for trans-fat. Here's a quiz question to test your knowledge:

Which of the following is trans-fat or contains trans-fat?
   a. Partially hydrogenated oil
   b. Shortening
   c. Margarine
   d. Coconut oil
   e. Only A, B and C
   f. All of the above

For those of you who chose option "E," you're exactly right! However, don't feel badly if you didn't choose the right answer because you'll learn more. Just keep reading!

For clarity, let's address what trans-fat is and why it's so harmful. Usually, natural fats are long chains of carbons and hydrogen atoms linked together. When there are simple, single bonds connecting all of the atoms in the fat, it's a saturated fat. Occasionally, when a double bond is present within the fat, it can change the chemical properties, e.g. monounsaturated fats (found in olive oil, canola oil, and safflower oil) or polyunsaturated fats (like in flax seeds, walnuts, or fish). When we consider oils containing double bonds more thoroughly, this is where trans-fat can be an issue. Normally, oils like soybean oil are liquids at room temperature. However, by adding hydrogen gas to the liquid oil, the mixture solidifies and the oil becomes less likely to go rancid.[34] This is what occurs during the hydrogenation process.

Although our bodies can tolerate and metabolize small amounts of naturally occurring types of trans-fat like those generally found in beef or lamb, the method of hydrogenating vegetable oil creates a slightly different type of trans-fat that must be metabolized in a different manner within our bodies. Despite the fact that this process saved big corporations lots of money by extending the shelf life of packaged foods, trans-fat was also causing a decline in consumer health.

Trans-fat contributes to negative changes in lipid profiles so low-density lipoprotein cholesterol (LDL-c) increases, and high-density lipoprotein cholesterol (HDL-c) decreases.[35] This is unfortunate because higher HDL cholesterol is generally associated with decreased risk of cardiovascular disease (CVD). This is because it is a dense form of cholesterol that can prevent the less dense forms from collecting on the walls of arteries kind of like a bowling ball knocking down idle, loitering pins that may eventually lead to blockages in blood vessels. To further complicate the matter, there are different types of LDL and HDL. As a result, some are more closely associated with CVD than others. There are blood tests that can differentiate which type of LDL or HDL cholesterol is elevated. You can ask your physician about ordering this special lab test for you.

Trans-fat can lead to insulin resistance also. You may be aware that insulin helps regulate blood sugar by helping to open cells so glucose can enter and provide energy. When a person shows signs of insulin resistance, it means their cells don't respond properly to glucose. So, the cells "resist" insulin's attempts to help the cells absorb glucose that is circulating throughout the blood stream. As a result, people may begin having high blood pressure, type II diabetes, arteriosclerosis, polycystic ovarian syndrome (PCOS), or metabolic syndrome.[36] Additionally, the extra glucose that's not used for energy is stored as fat, especially around the belly where it is typically not wanted.

Interesterified Oil

In lieu of increased consumer awareness and the inevitable, yet delayed, intervention of the FDA regarding the deleterious effects of trans-fat, manufacturers have sought comparable alternatives that wouldn't negatively alter taste or other sensations of processed foods. Thus, a new process has been adapted to modify vegetable oils making them similar to trans-fats without them actually being trans-fats.

The process of making interesterified oil is called interesterification, which involves breaking apart triacylglycerols (TAGs) into a glyceride molecule and three separate fatty acids.[37] This process involves the use of chemical catalysts like sodium methoxide or ethoxide, which must be removed via another chemical process.[38] Then, the fatty acids are reassembled back onto the glycerol backbone in an effort to produce a fat that is solid at room temperature with a higher melting temperature like butter that doesn't contain trans-fat like partially hydrogenated oil. This is where the process gets interesting: In order to decrease the chances that trans-fats are present, oil blends are interesterified with fully hydrogenated oil. Although only a small amount of hydrogenated oil may be used, the same toxic processes used for partially hydrogenated oil has furtively been eased into interesterified palm oil blends, palm kernel oil, and canola oil. At this point, labeling oils that are interesterified is not required. One study found that in comparison to partially hydrogenated oil, interesterified oils also altered metabolism of plasma lipoproteins (like LDL and HDL) and blood glucose in humans suggesting further research is necessary to officially accept interesterified oils as a better alternative.[39] As consumers, we should be aware.

Notably, there are some alternatives previously used in America that have withstood the test of time and have persistently been used in other countries where trans-fat is not permitted. Thus, consider using products that contain coconut oil, pure palm oil, and tallow. Contrary to what most people may think, saturated fats are not inherently bad. (This will be explained later.) In fact, certain fats may be what your body needs in order to feel satiated instead of carbohydrate rich foods you may often crave.

Omega-6 and Omega-3 Fatty Acid Imbalance
Although fat was addressed previously, there are other reasons to be concerned about how our industrialized mechanisms of

obtaining vegetable oils are altering normal processes in our bodies. For a moment, consider opposing and complementary things, e.g. what goes up must come down and what goes in must come out (perhaps in a different form). In organized systems, like our bodies maintaining homeostasis, or balance, there are opposing actions that keep everything functioning properly. A good physiological example of this is respiration. As oxygen levels are sufficiently maintained in the body through inspiration and expiration, our blood utilizes the available oxygen for respiration to keep the body functioning properly. However, if there is a decrease in oxygen available within our tissues, our bodies naturally accommodate and will begin hyperventilating to obtain more oxygen and breathe out excess carbon dioxide. This system of checks-and-balances works well to keep us breathing properly. Unfortunately, this process isn't as simple regarding dietary changes that have resulted in a different proportion of Omega-6 (n-6) fatty acids to Omega-3 (n-3) fatty acids.

Before the massive industrial transition that made vegetable oil readily available and cheap in industrialized countries, the average American had an Omega-6:Omega-3 ratio that was approximately 1:1, which essentially means there were 50 percent Omega-6 fats and 50 percent Omega-3 fats. Now, the ratio is tremendously weighed in favor of Omega-6 fatty acids between 10:1 and 20:1.[40] Research has demonstrated the imbalanced Omega-6:Omega-3 fatty acid ratio of is linked to neurodevelopmental deficits, decreased insulin sensitivity, psychiatric, respiratory, and cardiovascular conditions.[26,41,42] For this reason, this is generally an obstacle that must be addressed to restore health.

In their natural form, we would obtain Omega-6 fatty acids from oils found in animal products, nuts, seeds, grains (including corn), and cottonseed. In addition, we could obtain the proper balance of Omega-3 fatty acids from nuts, seeds (like flax and chia), green vegetables (like kale, purslane and spinach), and fatty fish (like wild salmon).[26] This would provide us with a good, balanced ratio of Omega-6:Omega-3 fatty acids.

In our bodies, these fats primarily aid in production of a variety of 20-carbon chain molecules collectively called *eicosanoids*. When functioning properly, they work as chemical messengers to increase or decrease the stickiness of platelets as needed, and they constrict or dilate smooth muscle in the lungs, blood vessels, and intestines. They also stimulate mucus production, inhibit cholesterol synthesis, and increase HDL (the good cholesterol). Within this system of checks-and-balances, different areas of the body utilize eicosanoid products like gamma linolenic acid (GLA), eicosapentaenoic acid (EPA), and docosahexaenoic acid (DHA) to keep our bodies functioning properly.

Since our bodies cannot produce essential fatty acids, the only way to correct the imbalance is to increase consumption of foods containing high amounts of Omega-3 fatty acids. Notably, partially metabolized Omega-6 from plant sources can be converted into arachidonic acid that increases inflammation. Although this conversion is relatively weak in humans, excessive consumption of packaged foods containing high amounts of soybean and corn oil may lead to more negative health consequences than once believed.

Finally, there are significant differences in the fatty acid composition of grain-fed animals in comparison to those that are pasture fed. Again, large-scale feedlots and production of animal products may also be contributing to the ratio imbalance. There is mounting research that demonstrates pasture fed cattle contain less total lipids and have a more balanced Omega-6:Omega-3 fatty acid ratio. These animal products also contain more antioxidants.[43] These are noteworthy differences in comparison to cattle from a feedlot, which is the source of most beef available in the United States. Since we can obtain a higher proportion of Omega-3 fatty acids from eating green vegetables in comparison to grains, metabolically, the same thing happens in cattle.

Hormones and Antibiotics in Animal Products
Mass production of animal products has posed other public health concerns. Food animals (i.e. animals raised for human consumption, dairy cows, and poultry producing eggs) have been routinely given antibiotics and hormones in an effort to hasten their maturation rate, to increase their size, and to prevent infectious diseases. As a result, products from such animals have increased our exposure to hormones and antibiotics. Unfortunately, excessive antibiotic use within the food animals industry has likely contributed to the increased the incidence of antibiotic resistant microbes.

Antibiotics:
Since the 1950s in the United States, antibiotics have been routinely used in the production of livestock intended for consumption. Typically added to food or water for the animals, the use of antibiotics in livestock serves dual purposes.

Surprisingly, the primary reason antibiotics have routinely been given to livestock is to expedite the maturation process of the animals while fattening the animals up. Although this effect improves "feed efficiency," the reason antibiotics have this effect on livestock is still poorly understood by scientists.[44] The process allows farmers to give the animals less food, which saves the ranchers and livestock growers money. Additionally, antibiotics can prevent infections from occurring in the farm animals.

Since antibiotics have been used frequently for such a long time, within the past several decades concerns regarding antibiotic resistance have emerged. In many feedlots for livestock and chickens, free-choice medicated feed (FCMF) is provided for the animals. As a result, the animals have the opportunity to feed as much as they desire. Unfortunately, this method of feeding the animals has yielded detrimental consequences. Some of the animals eat too much, and this leads to chemical toxicity in the animals and drug remnants in food.[45] One review analyzed many of the variable research attempts to recover quinolone residues within various animal food products. Although this is a complex process, many of the studies regardless of the method, recovered more than 60 percent of quinolones within the animal food product.[46] Since this was a review, it's unclear how much of the quinolones may have accumulated within the animals over time.

Additionally, constant low-dose exposure or even regular intermittent exposure of bacteria to antibiotics has provided an opportunity for bacteria associated with livestock and chickens to adapt to the antibiotics. Because of this, bacteria have developed antibiotic resistance genes that can be exchanged with other more virulent bacteria. This could result in pathogenic strains of bacteria being resistant to routine antibiotic treatment.[44] In Europe, bacteria with multiple drug-resistant traits were identified on nearby farms where antibiotics were not used on the animals. This finding demonstrates that the transfer of genetic resistance amongst microbes is relatively simple based on the interconnection of the ecosystem.[47] If we were wise, we'd consider such repercussions here in the United States.

Another effect of FCMF that impacts people who avoid consumption of animal products is related to *pharmacokinetics*. This term simply means how much of a drug is concentrated in circulation of an organism and how the drug is eliminated. The concern is that most types of antibiotics—75 percent—aren't even absorbed in the animals and are simply excreted. Thus, the drugs pass through them without being metabolized and enter the human food chain via rainwater runoff flowing to water treatment facilities and via fertilizer used from these animals for produce. Regardless of whether you eat animal products or not, there are still mechanisms of exposure to antibiotics in the environment as a result of how they have been used for decades.

In 2011, a group of health and consumer groups filed a lawsuit against the FDA demanding that action be taken based on the FDA's findings that antibiotic use in livestock increased antibiotic resistant bacteria. The FDA previously made an effort to "stop the use of 'extra label' that is unapproved use of cephalosporins, an antibiotic, in major species of food-producing animals such as cattle, pigs (swine), chickens, and turkeys."[48] In December 2013, the FDA informed the public that it is taking further steps to ensure the non-medicinal use of antibiotics will no longer be a common practice within three years time by "phasing out the use of medically important antimicrobials in food animals for production purposes (e.g. to enhance growth or improve feed efficiency)."[49] This change would require livestock growers to get prescriptions for sick animals from licensed veterinarians. It would also prevent pharmaceutical companies from labeling antibiotics in ways they were not originally intended to be used.

It seems the FDA is granting pharmaceutical companies time to determine if they will willingly comply with the transition and change the labeling of the antibiotics to only include use for disease prevention. The outcome will be interesting considering "the FDA reported that 13.1 million kilograms of antimicrobial drugs were sold or distributed for use in food-producing animals in 2009."[45] Notably, the FDA has been in communication with the American Veterinary Medical Association to ensure the laws regarding use of medically important antibiotics is conducted judiciously. However, strategies for monitoring and assessing implementation of the new law have yet to be revealed.[49,50]

Hormones:

Hormone use is another concern regarding livestock. "In 1993, the FDA approved the recombinant bovine growth hormone (rbGH), also known as bovine somatotropin (rbST), for use in dairy cattle to increase milk production."[51] An estimated 30 percent of U.S. cattle have been treated with rbGH. In addition, the FDA approved six different types of steroid hormones for use in U.S. food production. These hormones include estradiol, progesterone, testosterone, zeranol, trenbolone acetate, and melengestrol acetate. Zeranol, trenbolone acetate, and melengestrol acetate are synthetic growth promoters used to make animals grow faster. "Currently, federal regulations allow these hormones to be used on growing cattle and sheep, but not on poultry (chickens, turkeys, ducks) or hogs (pigs) since they are not as useful in increasing weight gain in poultry or hogs."[51] Notably, another synthetic estrogen called diethylstilbestrol (DES), was previously used in chickens but was phased out due to its association with cancer.

Just as antibiotics used in cattle eventually end up in water and soil, one research study also demonstrated the environmental effect of synthetic hormone use in livestock. For two years, researchers collected and analyzed 16 natural and synthetic hormones from runoff water, manure, and soil located in a feedlot with reasonably controlled conditions. Overall, the study primarily noted the main concern was that there were increased concentrations of hormones collected from areas where the cattle were treated with hormones. However, due to confined feedlot conditions, cattle treated with hormones as well as those that were not both experienced an overall negative environmental impact that has posed yet another public health concern.[52]

Numerous research endeavors have focused on the effects of hormones on humans. Consequently, there have been associations with increased rates of early and precocious puberty, hormone-related cancers, and male reproductive tract disorders, including undescended testicles in male babies and low sperm quality after puberty.[53] Many of the studies focus on endocrine disruptors and xenoestrogens, chemicals that exert similar effects as estrogen within the human body. Thus, there is necessity of research that focuses specifically on exogenous hormones introduced into the environment from raising cattle. One study that seemed to focus more in this area concluded that possible adverse effects from meat consumption of animals treated with exogenous hormones could not be excluded.[54] So, it's wise to err on the side of caution and limit consumption of products from animals that have likely been treated with hormones. This is particularly important during puberty and reproductive years.

High Fructose Corn Syrup

High fructose corn syrup (HFCS) is a man-made blend of fructose and glucose, which are *monosaccharides.* Monosaccharides are the simplest form of sugar that our bodies prefer to use for energy. However, in contrast to natural sugar like sucrose that is also comprised of one fructose and one glucose, HFCS lacks a chemical bond between fructose and glucose.[55] Therefore, the metabolic responses involving the pancreas, insulin and enzymes that typically assist with the breakdown of sugars does not occur. This skipped step in metabolism leads to rapid increases in blood sugar and overwhelms the liver with the responsibility of metabolizing excess simple sugar.[22]

Since the liver performs exponential tasks within the body, the liver adapts to the excess sugar from HFCS consumption by storing the sugar for use later. Although this is a logical use of the extra calories, the extra fructose is altered by the liver in a manner that can be stored in your body as fat—the crazy, not-so-sexy fat—that hangs around the midsection of your body.[56]

In biochemical terms, an enzyme called hexokinase phosphorylates the excess fructose. (Phosphorylation is the addition of three oxygen atoms attached to a phosphate atom that binds to another molecule as a group.) In its phosphorylated form, fructose becomes glyceraldehyde-3-phosphate, which then can be used in the synthesis of fats. In high amounts, HFCS contributes to increased adipose tissue. Many research endeavors support this association.[22,55]

Most people without underlying health obstacles who give up most processed foods containing HFCS naturally experience weight loss. It's also worth mentioning that weight gain is not always the undesired effect of HFCS consumption. Increasing rates of insulin resistance, hypertension, inflammation, and kidney or liver damage may also be associated with the copious amounts of HFCS Americans consume regularly.[57] Finally, there was an opposing view that many of the ideas surfacing regarding HFCS are unfounded particularly regarding the imbalanced ratio of glucose to fructose causing a metabolic problem.[58] Unfortunately, since so many other resources validate the skewed metabolic processes as a result of HFCS consumption, it's more reasonable to use caution and limit intake until other information is available. The FDA has taken a neutral stance on the matter as well and simply advises Americans to "limit consumption of all added sugar."[59]

Genetically Modified Organisms (GMO)
According to the United States Census Bureau, just over 300 million people live in the United States, and there are currently more than 7 billion people on the planet. As a result, ample food is necessary to sustain our rapidly growing population.

Unfortunately in many areas around the world, starvation is *still* a problem. In response to the growing demand for food, scientists and farmers have been working together to determine ways to supply food for our ever-increasing population. One controversial solution is genetically modified organisms (GMO).[60] According to Harvard School of Public Health, GMO products may also be called *genetically engineered* (GE) or *transgenic* foods.[61] *Biofortified* products may also be genetically modified, but the term has been used by non-GMO supporters who grow produce in enriched soil and by corporations that use biotechnology, the process of genetic engineering, to supposedly increase nutrient content in food. Currently, manufacturers in the U.S. are not required to label GMO products, but knowing the different aliases may be helpful. Although you may not have been aware of it as a U.S. citizen, "70 percent of the food products on your supermarket's shelves may contain ingredients from a biotech (or GE) crop and has been an everyday part of consumers' lives for the past 10 years."[62]

According to the World Health Organization (WHO), GMO products are "organisms in which the genetic material has been altered in a way that does not occur naturally."[63] Thus, some of the genes in the genetically modified organism have been artificially transferred into its genome to display traits and characteristics that were not originally present. Apparently, this process is quite haphazard and may affect other genes in the organism, especially since much of the DNA is used repeatedly to produce different proteins as described previously. Some of the most common types of genetic modifications implemented thus far include herbicide resistance, herbicide tolerance, and insect resistance.[64]

By conferring herbicide resistance within the genome of a specific plant, GMO supporters expected fewer chemicals would be needed to protect crops. In addition, this could decrease farmers' chemical exposures as well as consumers by decreasing the overall amount of herbicide in the environment. Unfortunately, a comparison study on cotton in China demonstrated there was no difference in the amount of pesticide used on the GMO cotton versus natural cotton since there was a sharp rise in secondary pests targeting the GMO cotton.[65] During a GMO Free Arizona presentation, a farmer who witnessed the effects of GMO products on the environment and the agricultural industry believes that even more chemicals are used on GMO crops to activate the inserted genes thus further increasing toxins within the environment as well as consumer exposure. A review of the report released in February 2014 by the USDA Department of Agriculture further supported his claim by noting that although insecticide use has decreased, herbicide use has increased and has resulted in more weed resistance.[66]

Another concern regarding GMO products is the potential drift of genetic material into non-GMO crop fields.[67] Simply stated, a "change in the wind" has led to adulterated organic products with undesirable GMO traits. As a result, there have been numerous legal disputes between farmers and biotechnology companies regarding contamination of non-GMO crops. There are also other issues related to ownership of such crops regardless of where the intentionally mutated genetic crops grow.

One gene that confers insect-resistance is the *cry* gene from a bacteria. When an insect consumes GMO crops with this inserted gene, an enzyme is created in the insect's mid-gut that form holes within the cell membranes of the cells lining the bug's gut. This rapidly increases the flow of fluids into the cells causing them to burst killing the cell and inevitably the insect. Although a protein transcribed from this gene, Cry9c, was not originally intended for human consumption, small amounts were found in corn products in Europe and have been linked to increased allergies.[64] From a naturopathic medical perspective, consumption of GMO proteins may also cause increased food sensitivities that are subtle irregular immune reactions to foods that may cause a myriad of symptoms like poor digestion, persistent nasal congestion, or even brain fog. Despite insufficient implication of the Cry9c protein following investigations based on consumer complaints, increased public concern about the potential health repercussions of GM food have risen tremendously since the first transgenic foods became available in the U.S. in the 1990s.

Since DNA is essentially comprised of the same molecules that are arranged differently in every living organism, there has also been growing concern about the safety of GMO foods using promoters that are essentially plant retroviruses. (A retrovirus is an infectious agent that inserts its genetic material within the DNA of a host organism to create replicas of the original virus.) The CaMV35Spro gene from cauliflower is a promoter that can lead to overexpression of certain genes and has been used in a variety of plants. In humans, retroviruses have been linked to human diseases, such as schizophrenia and even certain kinds of cancer.[64] For this reason, there is concern about GMO promoter DNA sequences potentially mingling with our DNA. The review also pointed out that about 10 percent of cabbage and cauliflower contain the CaMV plant retrovirus, so we've been exposed to this genetic sequence for some time now in these plants. Apparently, the GM foods with these promoter regions contain far less of the CaMV35Spro than the cabbage and cauliflower naturally containing the sequences. However, since GM products from corn and soy tend to be quite abundant in many processed foods, repeated exposure may be an issue.

Another concern based on GM foods is nutrient density. One study demonstrated 12 to 14 percent less isoflavones in GM soy with glyphosate herbicide resistance. In opposition, there were other studies demonstrating variability in isoflavones content in GM soy compared to conventional types. In these studies, nutrient density was more closely associated with environmental factors.[64]

According to the National Research Council, GMO products are likely to result in an "unintended adverse effect."[68] The reason for this outcome is based on basic principles of ecology. For example, suppose there is a group of organisms, let's say pea plants, and most of these pea plants were offspring from one common ancestor. In this case, there is minimal genetic variety or variability amongst the group as a whole and future populations will likely be stable. In contrast, when mutations are induced within the population of pea plants, this disrupts the originally stable gene pool by introducing unknown genes. These genetic mutations are "most likely to display unintended effects from the widest potential range of phenotypic effects." This means that in addition to variable physical attributes of the GMO generation of pea plants, the probability of something else being different based on the plants new gene sequence is relatively high, and it would be difficult to predict the "unintended effects." Perhaps in response to this information, another research study concluded that "unintended effects may have positive, negative, or indeed no consequences on the agronomical vigor or safety profile of the crop."[69] This article also mentioned that "unintended effects" may occur in non-GMO crops as well but aren't required to undergo as many safety assessments. Again, there are numerous conflicting perspectives regarding the overall effect of GMO product consumption, especially since these products have only recently been introduced to consumers within the last 20 years.

In January 2014, various consumer interest groups, businesses, and some congressional leaders, held a press conference regarding a letter they were submitting to President Barack Obama reminding him about his campaign pledge to require GM foods to be labeled. Some of the groups supporting the cause included the Environmental Working Group, the Center for Food Safety, and Just Label It.[70]

There have also been attempts in some states to get bills passed that would require suppliers to inform consumers if a particular product has been genetically engineered. Unfortunately, limited funding has continued to stifle efforts of organizations in favor of transparency, while big businesses like Monsanto hold patents for many of the GM crops used in foods and continue to control the political forecast in opposition to labeling GM foods. Some of their campaigns lead consumers to believe that labeling GM foods would lead to an increase in prices.[71]

Currently, some of the most common GM products that are widely available include[72,73]:

• Corn	• Canola	• Rice
• Soy	• Sugar beets	• Tomatoes
• Zucchini		• Potatoes
• Yellow Crookneck Squash	• Cotton	• Peas
	• Papaya	• Atlantic Salmon*
	• Alfalfa	

*An FDA authorization request for GMO Atlantic salmon was submitted in 2008; Inserted genetic sequence allows salmon to grow twice as fast, but lacks nutrient density compared with non-GMO salmon; Canada approved production of GMO salmon eggs in November 2013.[74, 75]

Based on this list, the typical American probably gets most dietary GMO product exposure from products like high fructose corn syrup, soybean oil, canola oil, and sugar.

Since there have been growing concerns regarding the safety of GM foods and their potential impact on the health of the consumer, many other countries have banned GM foods due to the uncertainty of the consequences and repercussions from long-term consumption of these products. Consumers must remain well informed and choose foods wisely. Research has linked GMO products to decreased food quality, antibiotic resistance, toxicity, allergenicity, accidental gene transfer to non-GMO crops, creation of new viruses and toxins, and threatened crop diversity.[65]

GMO products also raise religious, cultural, ethical, and environmental concerns that may warrant avoiding such products. One way to potentially avoid consumption of GM foods is to buy organic varieties that are commonly genetically engineered. Since it is illegal in the United States for a product to be labeled organic if it is genetically modified, you can avoid foods that most likely contain transgenic ingredients and choose the organic versions instead. The price look up (PLU) number of organic produce will have a "9" preceding four other numbers.[76] Although not required by the FDA, some GMO produce may have an "8" preceding other four numbers.

Consumers can identify packaged organic foods by looking for the black and white or green and white "USDA Organic" label. Alternatively, you can look for the black and white "Quality Assurance International Certified Organic" label. A non-profit organization called the Non-GMO Project independently tests products to determine if GMO ingredients are present in packaged foods. If products pass their standardized verification process, the product can have the Non-GMO Project verification mark, which is an orange butterfly on a leaf, on the packaging. This doesn't imply the item is organic, but supports that the ingredients are not made from GM foods.

Preservatives & Food Additives

Companies producing packaged foods have generally aimed to keep costs low and as a result unfortunately add ingredients that are not beneficial for consumer health. In a similar manner as partially hydrogenated oil, which was addressed previously, a myriad of other preservatives and chemicals have been added to foods to preserve or extend shelf life. Some ingredients have been added to packaged foods for aesthetic effects adding color or scent to foods. Other additives have also been included to produce a neurological response that increases the consumer's desire for that particular food.

Unfortunately, many of these chemical preservatives have other known consequences from consumption. In the U.S., many carcinogens (substances that promote cancer growth) are permitted within the food supply. Although limits may be placed on the amounts of these substances included in food, it's still disconcerting that certain chemicals that are "generally recognized as safe" are even allowed in food. Some of the culprits include: butylated hydroxyanisole (BHA), calcium disodium ethylenediaminetetraacetic acid (EDTA), trisodium phosphate, brominated vegetable oil (BVO), tertiary butylhydroquinone (TBHQ), disodium guanylate, sodium benzoate, sulfites, and methylene chloride. A few will be addressed in this section. However, it's most important that you are aware of potential effects of additives in the foods that you consume regularly and that you strongly consider making adjustments.

Nitrates & Nitrites

Nitrates and nitrites are chemical compounds used to preserve certain foods. Nitrates can chemically become nitrites once exposed to saliva. In general, nitrites are typically used as preservatives in processed meats like hot dogs, bacon, pastrami, salami, pepperoni, ham, deli meats, and hamburgers. Meat preparation typically involves either smoking the meat or adding salt or other chemicals to it.[77] This process also may be done with certain cheeses. Once consumed, nitrites combine with amines (organic molecules already contained in the food) and are metabolized into *N*-nitrosamines, which were known carcinogens in humans.[78]

Based on this association, there have been numerous negative claims proposed about human consumption of nitrates and nitrites. The American Institute for Cancer Research supports the following assertion: "People who eat red meat should consume less than 500g (18oz) a week, and very little if any should be processed." This amount is equivalent to eating approximately three cooked, fist-sized servings of meat each week. Based on these guidelines, it seems wise to use caution when consuming processed meats or even cheese.

In contrast, recent data presents an opposing view supporting that consumption of nitrates and nitrites may actually be beneficial in lieu of their potential to generate increased amounts of nitrous oxide, NO. Nitrous oxide is a potent vasodilator that has notably had positive effects like decreasing blood pressure in hypertensive patients, decreasing inflammation, and protecting heart cells after a heart attack.[79,80]

Thus, based on variable opinions, moderation, or complete avoidance is best since NO can be produced via other mechanisms. Notably, vitamin C can also reduce formation of *N*-nitrosamines created from nitrate and nitrite consumption presenting yet another reason supporting that regular consumption of vegetables and fruits can help prevent many long-term negative health consequences.

Monosodium Glutamate

Monosodium glutamate (MSG) is comprised of glutamate, an amino acid, and a sodium atom. Gaining widespread acceptance in the U.S. in the mid-1900s, MSG, originally sold as

Accent, was declared a food that is "generally recognized as safe."[81] Unfortunately, it doesn't seem to be safe for some subsets of the population who react negatively after consumption of the substance. Previously linked to "Chinese restaurant syndrome," MSG was found to cause symptoms such as headache, numbness, flushing, tingling, palpitations, and drowsiness.[82] Other adverse effects linked to MSG consumption include obesity, depression, and eye damage.[81]

One of the main health concerns associated with MSG consumption is neurotoxicity also known as *excitotoxicity*. This process causes decreased oxygen availability for neurons, and in the brain low oxygen levels may lead to brain injury.[83] This research conducted in the 1990s associated MSG with ischemic events that potentially compromised the health of nerve cells. One recent study found extracts from *Calendula officinalis* (a flowering plant) were protective against oxidative stress and excitatory brain damage.[84] Again, countering negative effects of chemical additives with plants or products from plants seems to be advantageous.

It's also important to be aware of other names of ingredients that contain MSG that may be in foods you consume. The FDA notes that "MSG occurs naturally in ingredients such as hydrolyzed vegetable protein, autolyzed yeast, hydrolyzed yeast, yeast extract, soy extracts, and protein isolate as well as in tomatoes and cheeses."[82] Additionally, other ingredients that may contain MSG or produce MSG during processing include natural flavor, natural flavorings, seasonings, soy sauce, soy protein, maltodextrin, citric acid, carrageenan, enzymes, or enzyme modified ingredients.[81] In summary regarding MSG, if you happen to be sensitive to the substance, it is wise to avoid it, and talk to your doctor about using *Calendula* whenever you eat out at restaurants. However, if you're not MSG sensitive, moderation is still wise for a proper nervous system function.

BHA & BHT

Butylated hydroxyanisole (BHA) and butylated hydroxytoluene (BHT) are artificial antioxidants used commonly as preservatives in food and beauty products.[85] In food, BHA and BHT prevent rancidity and maintain the crispiness of products to extend shelf life. Manufacturers also add these chemicals to potato chips, chewing gum, cereal, candy, enriched rice, Jell-O, and vegetable oils to prevent flavor or color change of food.[86] BHA and BHT have been associated with chronic urticaria, or red, often round and itchy welts that persist on the skin. Although one study showed that low doses of BHA and BHT were not significantly associated with stomach cancer, some concern exists regarding the potential of BHA to be changed chemically into TBHQ, which is associated with producing reactive oxygen species (ROS).[87] "ROS have been implicated in events that have been associated with tumor promoting activity as well as the initiation of cell proliferation." Thus, consumption of BHA and BHT should also be minimal or avoided completely.

Aspartame

Some packaged foods and beverages along with most chewing gums contain a low-calorie artificial sweetener called aspartame. Yes, more than likely, the piece of gum you just had earlier contained aspartame. (You could check now.) Also, you likely have seen artificial sweetener packets on your table at restaurants. Those blue and pink packets are often used to sweeten coffee or tea. Aspartame is 180 times sweeter than regular table sugar and apparently doesn't affect blood sugar negatively.[88,89] Unfortunately, there are other potential negative health problems associated with it. Aspartame has been linked to irregular immunological responses resulting in the conglomeration of various white blood cells.[90, 91] This may pose a problem because "loitering" white blood cells can't fight infections! Another issue with aspartame is how the body metabolizes it. Aspartame is changed into methanol, which is later converted to formaldehyde in the body. Notably, "the International Agency for Research on Cancer (IARC) classifies formaldehyde as a human carcinogen. In 2011, the National Toxicology Program named formaldehyde as a known human carcinogen in its *12th Report on Carcinogens*."[92] Despite this known connection, the EPA only considers aspartame detrimental in high amounts or after prolonged exposure. If it is used regularly as a substitute for sugar, then this should be considered prolonged exposure that may cause cancer. Be aware of the potential outcome before repetitively reaching for the little sugar-substitute packages to sweeten your favorite beverage or even to freshen your breath with chewing gum. Though it may seem minor, your artificial sweetener or gum chewing habits could lead to health problems if unaddressed.

Azodicarbonamide

Azodicarbonamide, an asthma triggering allergen, is an ingredient used to bleach flour in bread and cereal. It is banned in Australia, the United Kingdom, and many European countries. "Up to 45 parts per million is considered safe in the U.S., and it's found in a wide range of breads and baked goods."[93] Azodicarbonamide gained negative attention after a petition against SUBWAY® Restaurants highlighted that the ingredient used in many of the breads available on the menu is also used in yoga mats as a foaming agent.[94] Apparently, SUBWAY® agreed to remove the chemical from the bread at some point in the future. The FDA has apparently continued to research the health effects associated with consumption of this ingredient. In particular, once combined with water, azocarbonamide forms semicarbazide, which is a concern because in rat studies it has been shown to increase the incidence of tumors in female mice.[95] Another recent rat study demonstrated potential liver toxicity associated with semicarbazide.[96] Again, it's important to be cognizant of what is permitted in the food here in the U.S., especially since this particular ingredient isn't even necessary to make bread! (Be mindful that in the "science world" lab rats are often used during experiments for ethical reasons since humans surprisingly have similar genes and metabolic processes. Research is then conducted with consenting humans when the experiments seem relatively safe for lab rats.)

Artificial and Natural Flavors

Have you ever read the list of ingredients for a food you had considered purchasing or were about to consume and saw *artificial flavorings* or *natural flavorings* listed? Did you wonder what these ingredients really were? The answer to this question is best addressed by stating what they are not. According to the FDA, artificial flavor means any substance used to impart flavor that "is not derived from a spice, fruit or fruit juice, vegetable or vegetable juice, edible yeast, herb, bark, bud, root, leaf or similar plant material, meat, fish, poultry, eggs, dairy products, or fermentation products thereof." In contrast, natural flavor or flavoring "means the essential oil, oleoresin (oil plus resin), essence or extractive, protein hydrolysate, distillate, or any product of roasting, heating, or enzymolysis, which contains the flavoring constituents derived from a spice, fruit or fruit juice, vegetable or vegetable juice, edible yeast, herb, bark, bud, root, leaf or similar plant material, meat, seafood, poultry, eggs, dairy products, or fermentation products thereof, whose significant function in food is flavoring rather than nutritional. Natural flavors include the natural essence or extractives obtained from plants listed."[97] So since that's *really* clear, it must be completely safe for human consumption... right?! Wrong! There are too many variations based on what the FDA allows to be classified as artificial and natural flavoring to the extent that consumers would be quite busy attempting to contact manufacturers to determine exactly what natural flavor means in this packaged food or what artificial flavor means in that beverage. Further, if health issues associated with a specific artificial or natural flavor arise, it may be difficult to pinpoint which products contain the flavoring that should be avoided. Limiting consumption or general avoidance may simplify the matter.

The Food Coloring Conundrum
Since people tend to associate certain colors with flavors, manufacturers use our natural associations with foods like red strawberries and orange oranges to simulate a familiar

experience with processed foods. Thus, many processed foods contain some dyes associated with the flavor of an item. As it turns out, brilliant blue (Blue #1) isn't so brilliant for our health! Allura red (Red #40), tartrazine (Yellow #5), and fast green (Green #3) also have negative associated health risks.[98] Some of these artificial colors are derived from petroleum,— the same material used to refine gasoline and diesel oil. Maybe that's why hyperactivity is a common side effect since it fuels kids' engines! Food dyes have also been associated with lymphomas and hyperactivity (Red #40, Yellow #5), DNA damage (Blue #1, Red #40, Yellow #5), bladder tumors (Green #3), and thyroid tumors (Yellow #5). Tartrazine has been extensively associated with allergies and asthma. It may also cause insomnia in some cases as well.

There have been efforts based on research to ban food dyes known to be particularly harmful to animals and humans. For example, erythrosine (FD&C Red #3) was delisted in the U.S. in 1990. However, there hasn't been any haste to remove it completely from consumer use.

> "This delisting was as a result of the Delaney Clause, which restricts the use of any color shown to induce cancer in humans or animals in any amount. However, erythrosine was not regarded as being an immediate hazard to health and products containing it were permitted to be used until supplies were exhausted."[99]

Considering other countries like Europe and Sweden have banned use of such additives in foods, perhaps collectively we need to ban foods containing these types of dyes and support manufacturers who use natural sources of food coloring. In lieu of this, look for products that contain "paprika, beet juice, carotene, red cabbage and turmeric" for coloring instead.[100]

Sodium Benzoate

Sodium benzoate was one of the first preservatives approved for use as an antimicrobial in foods by the FDA in the early 1900s.[101] However, in order to have antimicrobial properties desired for food preservation, sodium benzoate must lose its sodium atom to form benzoic acid. Benzoic acid occurs naturally in some foods particularly those that are acidic like some fruits and fermented products. Despite the slight variation in structure, sodium benzoate is commonly used as a preservative and could result in more harmful health effects.

For example, when sodium benzoate is combined with ascorbic acid (vitamin C), benzene may form. This is a concern because benzene is a carcinogen, a cancer causing substance.[101] There is also growing concern that products containing sodium benzoate may be exposed to ultraviolet (UV) light or heated during transit to a store to be sold. This exposure may potentiate benzene formation.

With high exposure, sodium benzoate can be quite toxic. For this reason, the FDA only permits a "maximum level of 0.1% in food."[102] However, it is also used in concentrations of 0.02 percent to 0.5 percent in oral medications (including some supplements), and 0.1 percent to 0.5 percent in cosmetics.[99] Since there are other rules for sodium benzoate concentration in pharmaceuticals and cosmetics, repetitive use and consumption of products containing the compound can increase exposure. In addition, sodium benzoate, like certain food dyes, has been implicated with increasing incidences of hyperactivity since it is commonly a preservative in fruit juices and soda.[103] Again, limiting exposure would be prudent.

Tainted Produce

Now, that you are seriously contemplating avoiding consumption of processed and packaged food, there's yet another concern. Much of the produce available in grocery stores may have been treated with chemical sprays or treatments that are fungicides, pesticides, colorants, or ripening/anti-ripening agents.[104] Unfortunately, there are no labels on produce to inform consumers if certain fresh fruits and vegetables were coated with chemicals, washed in water containing chemicals, or treated with chemicals in other ways during storage or transport. Many of these chemicals are documented as harmful substances, yet they are still used in the agro-industry. Here are some examples of chemicals that may be used on produce:

- Hydrazine compounds: These are used on produce to hasten ripening; commonly used on potatoes.
- Thiabendazole: This is a fungicide used on foods like bananas, apples, pears, and sugar beets to prevent or delay the appearance or growth of mold or fungus.
- Maleic hydrazide: This compound is used to prevent sprouting of root vegetables like potatoes, carrots and onions. It induces dormancy in citrus fruits.
- Sulfuryl fluoride: This compound is used as a fumigant on crops that are stored after harvest.

There have been efforts to ban the use of this particular substance since it's known to be neurotoxic.[105]

In addition to lowered IQ in children from exposure to sulfuryl fluoride, other potential health effects from these chemicals include toxic effects to the liver and thyroid,[106] blood,[107] and nervous system.[108] The EPA also notes that maleic hydrazine is known to induce cancer, yet continues to permit low concentrations to be used on foods.[109] For now, the following are viable solutions:

- Wash produce just prior to use with a diluted mixture of ½ cup of vinegar and 1 cup of water or diluted mild soap since waxy films tend to be oil based. [110]
- Purchase organic foods whenever possible, especially those consumed most frequently.
- Peel inorganic produce that tends to be most heavily coated with chemicals. Refer to the Environmental Working Group's "The Dirty Dozen" list each year.
- Consider rotating the types of produce you eat regularly based on the season and switch varieties (e.g. with apples use Fuji, Granny Smith, or Honeycrisp) at different times each year.
- With the guidance of a health care professional, consider cleansing or fasting annually for a brief period of time to allow your gastrointestinal system time to rest in an effort to decrease your total body burden from environmental exposures including toxins in and on food.

~

In conclusion, please don't be overwhelmed by the scientific and technical aspects of the information presented in this chapter. Instead, let's be careful not to tempt the Lord our God by consciously bombarding our bodies with an onslaught of chemicals and forms of food we were never intended to consume. Instead, let's be diligent and intentional about being aware of what is permitted during the production and processing of food in the United States. As Christians, let's run our race with diligence and consume foods in their natural form as much as possible. This alone will eliminate many of the potential negative effects associated with additives in processed foods. By doing so, instead of suffering from common chronic diseases, we can "be about our Father's business."[111]

Chapter Four: Renewing Your Mind

You are a spirit living in a body that has a soul comprised of your mind, will, and emotions.[112],[113] So, here's a question you should answer honestly: Which part of you determines what you eat every day? As children of God, it's important that we honestly address this question. Also, we must recognize that change may be necessary in order for us to walk in the fullness of God's promises to us regardless of how tormenting it initially may seem to refrain from consumption of some of our most beloved delicacies. Jesus came so that we might have life more abundantly.[5] Yet, if our consistently poor dietary choices made in the flesh sabotage God's promises, we will never experience the full life promised to us. This is how chronic, degenerative diseases ease into our lives.

Habits
Eating three meals daily tends to be the general consensus regarding how frequently we should eat. Not surprisingly, this may be challenging for most people since breakfast is exceptionally challenging to incorporate or at least to incorporate in a healthy manner for most people. For this reason, it is wise to determine if the frequency of your meals and snacks is helping to improve your health or if it's

functioning in an opposing manner. Additionally, it is also worth noting when your metabolism is able to manage digesting heavier meals. This varies for each individual.

Breakfast is truly the most important meal since the first meal generally sets the tone each day. Let's do a comparison of breakfast options: Breakfast A is comprised of a doughnut and coffee, and Breakfast B is comprised of a baked frittata with broccoli, bell peppers, and mushrooms with a half of an avocado.

Breakfast A happens to be full of sugar, which causes a rapid spike in blood sugar. In response, the pancreas has to produce sufficient insulin to control the excessive sugar levels. Shortly thereafter, blood sugar levels drop sharply which often leads to symptoms like grogginess, irritability, and cravings for even more sugar. The person eating Breakfast A also has caffeine triggering a sympathetic, or fight-or-flight response in the body. With the body on high alert as a result of the caffeine, the person's liver must work harder to metabolize the caffeine and convert the excess sugar from the doughnut into fat since there's an abundance of extra sugar in the body.

In contrast, Breakfast B tends to render altogether different metabolic results. First, the egg in the frittata is a complete protein. Protein does not spike blood sugar and is metabolized in a manner that does not lead to fat storage. The veggies provide additional nutrients in the form of vitamins and minerals coupled with fiber. Additionally, the avocado contains healthy fats, like Omega-3 fatty acids and vitamin E, which actually slow down digestion and keep the consumer satiated much longer. Thus, a person eating Breakfast B would probably not be hungry again until lunchtime.

Based on the comparison, it's important to set yourself up for success by being aware of how breakfast can help improve your health. In contrast, it may also be one of the main reasons you're not as healthy as you'd like to be. Skipping breakfast is also not a wise option because making this a regular habit can lead to a decreased metabolic rate and stunt weight loss. Eating the right types of foods earlier in the day actually jump-starts your metabolism helping you burn calories more efficiently throughout the day. Waiting to eat until lunchtime or in the evening typically slows metabolic function, and this is not favorable if weight loss is one of your goals. Most people tend to eat a rather large lunch or dinner as a result of skipping breakfast. If you simply aren't hungry in the morning, consider eating less at night or avoiding eating three to four hours before going to sleep.

Lunch proposes other challenges that can compromise many health goals, particularly due to peer pressure. If you work in an office or other setting where going out to a restaurant for lunch is typical, you probably can relate to peer pressure. Though you can choose healthier options at restaurants, most provide hefty servings of food that can also cause your blood sugar to spike with insulin and fat storage following suit. For this reason, it may be a better idea to pack your own lunch in order to save money, control portion sizes, and consume foods that help you maintain a healthy weight. Of course, preparation is typically dreaded and causes most people to default back to their old habits, but setting the intention and being disciplined in this arena can improve your results. Try taking your lunch just one day each week to begin. Over time, you can address any obstacles and increase the frequency of taking your lunch to work. You can be successful at this. As it relates to your social life in the office being compromised, try convincing your peers to order take-out so you all can eat together at a local park or just go out with them to eat one or two days each week instead of every day. Use your influence to help shake up how things have typically been done. Once others see your health improve, they will want to be like you!

Now, about the third meal of the day... If you're like most Americans, dinner can occur in a rather haphazard fashion. For most people, dinnertime is centered on cramming in other extracurricular activities for you and the family. If this is the case, perhaps pre-meal planning and preparation are better options so dinner only needs to be warmed up. Since many foods freeze well after being cooked, you could try prepping meals for dinners throughout the week and freeze them. At the same time, you can prepare lunches and complete the huge task of food preparation in one 3-to-4-hour time block during the weekend or on other days you don't have to work. Additionally, if you have other family members living with you, work together completing the task and have some quality family time in the process. If you are financially able to do so, another option would be to hire a personal chef or subscribe to a healthy meal preparation service available in your area. This can free up about three hours weekly in your family's schedule and be well worth the investment. The overall point is to be intentional about eating a healthy, planned dinner instead of resorting to the "last-minute" hasty option of fast food or eating out frequently.

The time you eat dinner is also worth addressing. However,

it's important to point out a couple of things about sleep first. God designed our human bodies to require sleep. Many miraculous things happen during this process. Proper sleep helps you maintain a healthy weight and youthful appearance, decreases stress hormones, and improves immune and sexual function. All of these processes occur automatically to some degree when you sleep through the night. However, the efficacy and extent of these processes can be limited due to a "self-imposed" delay. These processes are actually limited by digestion. If there is food still hanging out in your stomach or small intestines when you slip into a restful slumber, your body prioritizes breaking down the food you ate and assimilating it or storing it for energy later. For this reason, eating dinner earlier in the evening, around seven o'clock and then not eating anything else afterward can help improve how well your body is replenished during sleep. This phenomenon is easier to notice when a person is fasting or consuming fewer calories. Typically, people observing these practices don't need as much sleep after a few days. Again, this is because going to sleep with an empty stomach capitalizes on the restoration that occurs during sleep. For this reason, it may help to include some healthy fat and protein with dinner to ensure you won't feel hungry just before going to sleep. This strategy can also help you feel hungry when it's time for breakfast in the morning.

Finally, snacking tends to be a favorite pastime for many of us. Snacks are totally fine and can help keep your blood sugar from dropping too low if you get hungry between meals. However, snack quality and quantity should be considered. When are you most likely to reach for a snack? Do you tend to gravitate toward carbohydrate-rich snacks or others that are sweet, salty, fatty or a combination of sorts? When you come home, is it usually a good time to grab a snack? Does watching TV feel weird without munching on something? Do you only grab snacks when you're hungry? If you're a fertile lady, do you tend to eat more snacks just before your period begins each month? Do you typically carry a snack with you just in case you get hungry? Take some time to reflect on your habits and gauge how adjustments can be helpful. Using some of the same strategies noted previously for meals, planning ahead can help you pack healthy snacks that will improve your health and keep you satiated between meals.

Ideally, snacks should contain protein and fat as well, which makes nuts, seeds, boiled eggs, or even sardines ideal. If you digest dairy well, cheese is a reasonable choice too. Vegetables are also good options, because the extra fiber can help you feel full. Also, if it's close to the time of your next meal, having a piece of fruit is clever since fruit will digest easily and satiate you until it's actually time to eat. It's best to avoid packaged snack foods as many contain excess sugar, salt, preservatives and unhealthy fats as previously addressed.

Food & Emotions

Since your soul is made up of your mind, will, and emotions, let's address what happens emotionally when you get ready to indulge in something that's not so healthy. There *it* is—the doughnut, the bag of potato chips, or the candy—the whatever *it* is that makes your mouth salivate and your heart palpitate! What emotion typically comes along with the experience leading up to partaking of your most beloved treat? Perhaps it's infatuation, jubilation, delight, bliss, or amazement. Yummy! The first bite is the best! Feels like heaven! Suddenly, neurotransmitters (chemical messengers) that make you feel happy become abundantly available in your brain as you eat this tasty treat bite after bite. You yearn to savor the last bite before your special beloved treat is all gone. Then, there are other emotions that follow consumption of the treat as well. Some people may experience satisfaction, relief, or comfort, while others may experience disappointment, disgust, guilt, or shame.

Experiencing emotions in your soul is not morally wrong. However, when an emotion leads or entices you to sin, this is when problems can manifest. There's a scripture that says, "In your anger, do not sin."[114] It seems that *any* emotion that triggers us to sin would not be pleasing to God. For this reason, take time to consider how different emotions lead you to behave as it relates to food. It may be extremely helpful to write this information down and look for patterns. When you feel frustrated, disappointed, or angry, do you self-soothe with food? When you feel overwhelmed or exhausted, do you grab the nearest carbohydrate-rich snack or drop by the coffee shop to help you power through the lull? How do you respond to rejection, abandonment, or loneliness? Is food your initial source of comfort or do you honestly make an effort to seek the kingdom of God first?[115]

These questions are not intended to point out anyone's shortcomings as we've all been there. Neither is the goal to be judgmental about what you do when things get challenging in life. However, the core issue that must be addressed is that our tendency to pacify ourselves with food *technically*

73

demonstrates a lack of self-control.[116] Take a moment to be realistic and transparent about the how the enemy is cunningly deceiving the body of Christ. We must demonstrate self-control in *every* area of our lives including something as simple as food.

Food, TV, and Boredom

Sometimes we eat because we're comfortably propped up in front of the television or reclined at a local movie theater. Regardless of our location, studies confirm an association with increased food consumption based on more food being available.[117] Intentionally making adjustments based on this wisdom can help spare us the over consumption of empty calories. So, if we aren't extremely hungry, we can opt for a bowl of our favorite snack as opposed to bringing the whole bag or box of the snack over to the couch with us to watch television. Also, ordering a small bag of popcorn or sharing a large bag at the movies may be wise as well.

On other occasions, being idle may lead us to eat more than we really need to or even want to. Although often associated with watching television or surfing the Internet, typically when people want to find something to do to fill the time, electronic devices are a quick, entertaining solution just like food! We ask ourselves, "Hummm, what can I do to make myself feel happy since I have some extra time?" Unfortunately, most of us don't opt for food choices that will help us feel good in *both* the short-term and long-term. In 2011, the CDC reported that only 20.6 percent of adults met basic guidelines for aerobic and muscle-strengthening physical activity.[118] So, it seems most of us opt to chill out watching something for entertainment perhaps subconsciously nibbling on whatever our flesh favors in the moment. However, as the body of Christ, we worship by the Spirit of God and glory in Christ Jesus and put no confidence in the flesh. Thus, when we have moments of reprieve, let's use wisdom to not allow our flesh to dictate the outcome.

Serotonin: Eating Due to Cravings & Stress

One neurotransmitter that is associated with "happy" feelings is serotonin, formally known as 5-hydroxytryptamine or 5-HT. Interestingly, most serotonin is produced in the gastrointestinal tract.[119] Special cells lining your intestines utilize the amino acid tryptophan to make serotonin. Once produced, it is shipped in transporters that take serotonin to a deeper level within the layers of cells lining the intestines where nerve terminal receptors await its release. Once released, the person experiences an immediate sense of comfort. Unfortunately, this mechanism may cause us to resort to consuming sweets and carbohydrate-rich foods to repeatedly experience this feeling of comfort—kind of like an addiction. Many studies also support the idea that low levels of serotonin could be associated with depression. In such cases, it is believed that there is an insufficient uptake of tryptophan leading to inadequate production of serotonin.[120]

Notably, there are other biochemical causes of depression as well. High levels of stress may result in increased use of serotonin throughout the body as an adaptive response.[121] Although most serotonin receptors are in the gastrointestinal (GI) tract, many other serotonin receptors are found throughout the body, particularly those associated with organs like the brain and adrenal glands that help us adapt during stressful situations.[122] Although researchers are debating the specific role of serotonin during stress, the presence of the receptors in certain locations in the body helps us recognize why eating sweets and carbohydrates seems to help us temporarily feel better during stress.

Hormonal Hunger: Ghrelin and Leptin

Guess what? There are also hormones associated with food cravings and our tendencies to either overeat or feel satiated. Ghrelin is a hormone produced in the stomach that is secreted when the stomach is empty. This generally starts about three to four hours after our last meal. On the contrary, leptin is produced by fat cells once we've eaten to signal to our brains that we should stop eating.

Scientific understanding of these hormones and their association with metabolism and natural rhythms between hunger and satiation is essentially in its infancy stages of our understanding. However, there have been some research endeavors aimed at determining if there are patterns that may affect our eating habits. One study compared how ghrelin levels were altered in non-diabetic patients compared to patients with type II diabetes. The study showed that in lean, non-diabetic participants, levels of ghrelin (the hunger signaling hormone) decreased significantly once leptin (the satiated signaling hormone) and insulin levels rose shortly after eating. In the obese participants, however, the amount of ghrelin was not suppressed leaving these individuals more likely to continue eating based on the hormonal imbalance.[123] Another study actually found leptin levels were higher in people with metabolic syndrome, which is a complex metabolic disease usually involving insulin resistance, abnormal lipids, hypertension, weight gain, and increased risks of clotting.[124] This was probably because the people in the study with metabolic syndrome had more fat cells to produce leptin. However, it may demonstrate how normal hormone fluctuations associated with eating can be altered in response to prolonged elevated levels of blood sugar leading to irregular metabolism and increased associated health risks. Finally, another study conducted on healthy young males correlated increased levels of ghrelin with decreased hours of sleep (less than four hours) per night over a three-day period. It was particularly notable that the types of foods desired during the sleep-deprived state included those that were rich in carbohydrates including "sweets, salty foods, and starchy foods."[125] Participants craved these carbohydrate-rich snacks 33 to 45 percent more than they did after adequate sleep of about nine hours though their desire for vegetables, fruits, and proteins was not as notable.

Considering this information, it's worth determining if appetite control issues are actually due to a hormonal imbalance. There are simple blood tests that can be performed to determine if this is an issue for you. If hormones are a factor, this awareness can help you and your doctor choose treatment options that can significantly improve your health.

Mind Over Matter

We have known for quite a while now that a person can alter their behavior simply based on their thoughts. "For as he thinks in his heart, so is he."[126] For this reason alone, it's imperative to be reflective about your thoughts regarding foods, and take control of your mind. Don't allow the enemy or even your own negative thoughts to make you feel as if you are missing out on something by eating a healthy diet regularly. Doughnuts, chips, or whatever you crave will be available tomorrow, next week, next month, and next year. However, your health status tomorrow, next week, next month, and next year will be based on how well you've trained your mind to recognize that healthy choices today are an investment in health both now and in the future. Eventually, you can have your favorite treat just not with the same frequency you've had it before. Also, "don't think physical food can satisfy the longing of your soul. Only Jesus can do that."[127]

What do you feel when you hear the words *broccoli* or *Brussels sprouts*? Is there a sense of distaste, disgust, or discomfort? Is there a feeling of rebellion since you were forced to eat the "little trees and cabbages" as a kid? If you have a negative association or reaction (excluding anaphylaxis from legitimate allergies) to these vegetables or any other type of vegetable or fruit, you must make some effort to reprogram your mind in order to successfully change your diet to include healthy, life-supporting foods. Be encouraged that your perspective regarding these types of foods can change, even to the point where you crave these healthy foods instead of the sugary sweets or salty delights you typically crave. One study demonstrated that preschool-age kids increased their intake of vegetables with a little bit of guidance.[128] Since you have the same power that raised Jesus from the dead at work in you, even your dislike of vegetables can be conquered! You can eat "rabbit food" and enjoy it!

When reflecting on our mentality regarding diet and

lifestyle, it's also important to recognize any cultural associations and beliefs you may have adapted as truths based on your formative years or any time afterward when you were highly impressionable. Reflect on the dietary habits that you may have adopted from your mother and father. Think about your grandparents and how they prepared their food. Are you noticing any patterns of unhealthy dietary habits? Did they exercise regularly? If not, you can be the initiator of healthy habits in your family tree!

It's interesting how our environments significantly impact who we become. This may be why there are so many examples of people used by God in the Bible who left their families and comfort zones to embrace their purpose. People like Moses, Abraham, David, Joshua, Ester, and Ruth stepped away from what was familiar to them. Perhaps God, in His divine wisdom, was attempting to show us through their examples that oftentimes, in order to be sensitive to what God wants for us in many areas of our lives, we may be required to do things differently. A research study claimed that some people might identify with a social or ethnic group and adapt the overall perspective and majority view on health behavior.[129] Unfortunately, this can be detrimental to you as an individual if your social or ethnic group doesn't routinely participate in health-promoting behavior. Remember, as sons and daughters of God, our identity is in Him. We "are no longer foreigners and aliens, but fellow citizens with God's people and members of God's household."[130] As members in His family, we should look like Him displaying all of the characteristics of God, including having dominion over everything—even doughnuts and chips!

Neighborhood & Budget Barricades

Since there are locations dispersed throughout the U.S. that may not have fresh produce readily available for purchase, a bit more effort may be required to take the first step at implementing dietary changes. In contrast, healthy food choices may be available in your area, but in higher-priced grocery stores that are not the most cost effective for your current budget. Both of these situations can be obstacles when attempting to create new dietary and lifestyle habits. For this reason, this section provides strategies and suggestions to help nullify the excuses that inadvertently sabotage your health.

With a plethora of information available at your fingertips, doing research on the Internet can set you up for success no matter where you live. Try a variety of search terms that will increase the probability that you will find healthy and affordable food options near you. Some examples include, "Farmers Market (your city or zip code)," "health food stores," "affordable healthy food," "(your city) Co-op," or "affordable produce." Lots of links will appear and by clicking through several of them, you will likely be able to find locations where healthy food at affordable prices is available in your area. Generally, prices at farmers markets are less expensive than those at local grocery stores since the "middle-man" is not profiting from the exchange. You may also negotiate prices particularly if you plan to purchase a large amount of produce. These markets may not be open daily and might have certain rules for participating. However, as you endeavor to find new alternatives to obtaining healthy food, it will get easier. Just remain committed. A list of potential resources is also available at the end of this section.

People can definitely be good resources as well! Ask your friends, neighbors, or co-workers if they know any locations where affordable produce is available for purchase. Ideally, you could ask an alternative health care professional, personal trainer, or organic restaurant owner in the area. Regardless, don't hesitate to ask around. As you grow in wisdom from asking around, an understanding about obtaining healthy food on a budget can be found![131]

Another resource is the local newspaper or other local publications. You can purchase a printed copy or check the online edition. Depending on consumer demand for healthy living in your city, there may be a whole section in the local newspaper devoted to providing such information. If not, consider contacting the newspaper to suggest that they add a section. In addition, there may be local publications like *Natural Awakenings* that highlight Complementary Alternative Medicine (CAM) specialists while listing local resources for healthy living in one place. These publications are free and are usually available at health food stores and or in locations where alternative health care is offered.

Internet Resources:
Retrieved February 28, 2014

USDA: http://search.ams.usda.gov/farmersmarkets/
The USDA sponsors a webpage to search for Farmers Markets in or near where you live. (There are numerous websites that offer this feature that may have different information so try several in your area for a comprehensive list.) If all the markets

you find are far away from your home, it may be wise to consider starting a local community farm or an organic farm to support your area. For more information on organic farming, visit the following link:
http://rodaleinstitute.org/2014/transition-to-organic/

Organic Kitchen: http://www.organickitchen.com
Organic Kitchen is an "organic foods product, research and marketing company." This website provides a "one-stop-shop" approach to the dilemma of finding organic produce in your area. It lists links to other companies providing services either online or in your local area. You can find Internet links to restaurants, farms, cooking classes, and much more!

Door-to-Door Organics:
http://www.doortodoororganics.com
Door-to-Door Organics is a food delivery service company that provides healthy food options for people living in the northeast and mid-America, particularly in Missouri, Nebraska, and Colorado. By teaming up with local organic farmers, they deliver custom boxes of fresh organic produce to customers.

SPUD: https://www.spud.com/index.cfm
Sustainable Produce Urban Delivery (SPUD) is a company that offers free delivery of fresh organic produce as well. This company specializes in bringing fresh foods into urban areas where it may be more costly to obtain fresh, healthy foods. They provide service along the West coast, including Los Angeles, Seattle, and some Canadian cities as well.

Food Cooperatives:
http://www.cooperativegrocer.coop/coops/
A food cooperative, or co-op, is like a local members club where each member pays a fee to be a part of the group that collectively buys into getting bulk produce for the members at a cheaper price. This is a great option in areas where local or organic farmers want to provide food to families directly. There are many options available, and sign up is generally simple.

CSA: http://www.localharvest.org/csa/
Another option that is relatively similar to a co-cop is Community Supported Agriculture (CSA). This type of arrangement is similar because there are local and organic farmers offering produce on a regular basis. However, the difference in many cases is usually participants pay upfront for the entire season of harvest with the average price ranging from $300 to $400 for a 24-to-26-week period in the growing season.[132] In addition, some farms offer other foods in addition to produce like meat, eggs, and milk.

Online Health Store Alternatives
www.vitacost.com, www.luckyvitamin.com,
www.iherb.com, www.truefoodsmarket.com,
www.shoporganic.com, etc.
In the past, location was everything! Now with Internet ordering options, you can order most things you would normally purchase from a local health food store from an online supplier at competitive prices. Even if you do frequently visit a health food store in your neighborhood, you may be able

to save money by bulk ordering from these companies. They tend to offer great deals on shipping also!

Ethnic Grocery Stores: http://www.mnn.com/food/healthy-eating/questions/how-can-i-get-produce-for-cheap
Depending on the city where you live, there may be notable cultural diversity. If this is the case, you may find venturing into a grocery store catering to certain ethnic groups can provide cheaper food options. There may be some interesting and diverse foods available, but don't allow that to hinder your quest for healthy food. Although, you may look differently than everyone else in the store, if you smile and give your money in exchange for their products, they will like you! In addition, some ethnic grocery stores may offer special savings that can really add up!

Large Chain Supermarkets
Now that health has become more important to the general public, more large chain grocery stores offer "natural food" sections. Some of these sections have a wide selection of products coupled with sufficient produce options. If this is the case, a trip to your neighborhood grocery store may be the solution you are looking for. That's easy! However, natural and organic selections are dependent upon your neighborhood though. There must be a demand for such products in order for the items desired to be available to customers. For this reason, it is imperative to communicate with the grocery store manager and let them know what you would purchase as a customer. It may also help if you get your family and friends to make requests as well. Additionally, since larger chain grocery

store managers recognize the gradual increasing demand for healthy foods, there are often good deals available in these stores. When you go to these types of stores, know exactly what you're going to get so you won't be distracted by many of the typical food options you purchased previously that are not health promoting. Take a list and only buy what's on it!

Other ideas for buying healthy foods within your budget include[132,133]:

- Buy in bulk, especially for beans and grains.
- Buy produce in-season because food is fresher and cheaper.
- Buy preserved foods during the off-season, preferably frozen or dried foods.
- Freeze foods for later. When a good deal is available, freezing food for a period of time (no more than six months) can yield substantial cost savings. Notably, the lower the water content in the food, the better it will freeze causing it to taste great later. It's also a good idea to use the frozen items as supplements for larger dishes like casseroles or soups.
- Plant a garden. If you have space, decent soil, and ample sunlight, it could be well worth the experience and quite rewarding too!

Chapter Five: Guidelines for Optimal Health

<u>Mind over Matter Solutions</u>

Now that you're equipped with an arsenal of resources to make dietary changes that can improve your health, you may be wondering, "*How* am I actually going to get myself to eat foods that I really don't like?" It's good that you want to know! First, avoid making ugly faces at the food or even at the thought of it! As an experienced eater, choose food in a more elegant manner by considering the value and health benefits of the food. This is similar to how we should view people—not merely focusing on physical attributes, but seeking to know the content of their character.[134] The "character" of nutrients in vegetables and fruits can make us better, healthier people just like friends of noble character! Figure out which seasonings make most vegetables taste good to you and use them regularly. Garlic powder and onion powder with a dash of sea salt work wonders for most vegetables. For even more zest, try adding paprika, turmeric, cilantro, or basil. If you like things spicy, add a little ginger or cayenne pepper. You may also mix the veggies with other foods like chicken and rice with teriyaki sauce. Then as you become more accustomed to eating vegetables, you can gradually include more for added nutrient density.

"Your Body: Vitamin-ville"

Did you know that there are certain nutrients our bodies require in order to function properly that *must* come from our external environment? Yes, we need to eat nutrient-dense foods to maintain and sustain healthy bodies. These nutrients are formally known as vitamins. Since our bodies cannot make or create them, it is essential that we consume foods or take supplements to avoid having physiological symptoms associated with nutrient deficiencies. The following information provides a brief synopsis of these vitamins and their functions in the body as well as what happens if levels are low.[135,136] Before reading the list, please be mindful that this information is not intended to prompt you to start supplementing these nutrients. Because there are toxicity symptoms associated with certain nutrients in excess, consult a licensed naturopathic physician for appropriate recommendations based on your individual needs.

- **Vitamin A**: This nutrient, also known as retinol, is formed from beta-carotene. It improves vision (especially at night) and supports immune cells in certain areas of the body like the upper airway. It can be toxic at high doses, especially in women attempting to conceive.

- **Vitamin B1**: Also known as thiamin, this nutrient helps us digest and assimilate carbohydrates, fats, and protein. Deficiency of vitamin B1 can lead to a condition called beri-beri, which involves numerous neurological symptoms due to degeneration of nerve cells throughout the body.

- **Vitamin B2**: Usually listed as riboflavin, vitamin B2 also helps us metabolize carbohydrates and makes it easier for other biochemical reactions in the body to occur.
- **Vitamin B3**: Also called niacin, this vitamin also helps with a myriad of chemical reactions throughout the body and is essential for cells to function properly. Deficiency of this nutrient can lead to a condition called pellagra, which consists of three primary symptoms, i.e. dermatitis, diarrhea, and dementia.
- **Vitamin B5**: Oftentimes called pantothenic acid, this vitamin is part of a coenzyme, which helps enzymes start reactions without using excess energy. Thus, vitamin B5 plays an indirect role in energy production, proper fat metabolism, synthesis of heme (the main portion of hemoglobin in the blood), and amino acid catabolism. Although isolated deficiency of vitamin B5 is rare, low levels have been associated with delayed growth, hair loss, impaired immunity, and decreased adrenal glands (stress response glands) function.
- **Vitamin B6**: Also known as pyridoxine, vitamin B6 assists with numerous reactions in the body especially in the blood, nervous system, and skin. It's also involved with steroid hormones like testosterone, estrogen, and DHEA. Deficient amounts of Vitamin B6 may cause nervousness, insomnia, anemia, and poor immune function.
- **Vitamin B7**: Biotin, another name for vitamin B7, acts as an enzyme for reactions in the body that need extra carbon, oxygen, and hydrogen atoms. Biotin also

activates another enzyme for proper glucose metabolism. Though it's usually easy to get sufficient biotin from food, raw egg whites contain an ingredient called avidin that prevents the body from using biotin. Low levels of biotin can lead to scaly skin, alopecia, and high cholesterol.

- **Vitamin B9**: Primarily known as folate, vitamin B9 is involved in DNA and RNA synthesis. It also helps metabolize Vitamin B12. It is essential for proper nervous system development and function, which is particularly important for developing babies shortly after conception. Low levels of folate may lead to anemia, anxiety, or impaired immunity. Folate also helps with homocysteine conversion because elevated homocysteine levels have been associated with cardiovascular disease and miscarriage.

- **Vitamin B12**: Typically called cobalamin, vitamin B12 helps with DNA synthesis, red blood cell formation, and homocysteine metabolism. It also serves integral roles for proper immune and nervous system function. Low levels may cause anemia, neurological symptoms (like tingling and numbness in fingers and toes), memory loss, and decreased immune capacity.

- **Vitamin C**: Ascorbic acid, vitamin C, is involved in hormone, collagen, and amino acid formation. It also plays important roles in immune function and wound healing. Vitamin C also helps in the absorption of iron and is a crucial antioxidant in the body. Severe cases of Vitamin C deficiency may lead to scurvy, gingivitis, fatigue, and skin rashes. In children, low Vitamin C levels may also cause impaired bone growth.

- **Vitamin D**: Calcitriol, the active form of vitamin D, can actually be synthesized in our bodies if, and only if, we get sufficient exposure to sunlight. Unfortunately, since there are so many warnings about skin cancer risks associated with sun exposure, most of us intentionally avoid sunlight and, as a result, have low levels of vitamin D in our blood. (If you have never had your levels checked, it would be wise to ask your doctor about it.) Vitamin D is actually like a hormone based on how it's formed and how it does different things throughout the body. It has a myriad of functions like enhancing calcium absorption, influencing cellular growth and development, preventing infections and autoimmune diseases, and enhancing insulin activity. The most familiar consequence of low levels of vitamin D is impaired bone mineralization, which may lead to rickets in children and osteomalacia (soft bones) and osteoporosis in adults. Recent research has compelled many medical doctors to recognize the importance of assessing vitamin D levels in patients.

- **Vitamin E**: Alpha tocopherol is the main form of active vitamin E in the body. Like vitamin C, vitamin E is an antioxidant that also has anti-inflammatory properties and assists in helping cell membranes to function properly. It also inhibits platelets from sticking together and has an enhancing effect on the immune system at appropriate doses. Vitamin E deficiency has been associated with muscle wasting and neurological degeneration. Clinically, Vitamin E may be useful for a myriad of conditions like atherosclerosis, scleroderma, sickle-cell disease, hepatitis, muscle cramps, painful periods, and infertility.

- **Vitamin K**: Menaquinones, different forms of vitamin K, help with clot formation in the body at appropriate times. Without sufficient vitamin K, in severe cases, a person could bleed to death without immediate intervention. More commonly though, mild vitamin K deficiency may result from inflammatory bowel diseases that compromise nutrient absorption in general. Dark green, leafy vegetables are abundant sources of vitamin K. In addition, sometimes bacteria in our gastrointestinal systems can produce vitamin K. Vitamin K may be recommended for ischemic heart disease, nausea and vomiting of pregnancy, and bleeding diseases in newborns. Interestingly, vitamin K also plays a role in bone health. For this reason, vitamin K_2, a specific form, is often helpful for osteoporosis.

There are also numerous minerals that serve important roles for health and proper function even though only small amounts of minerals are necessary. Some key minerals and their functions are noted below:

- **Calcium**: As an integral structural component of bones and teeth, calcium is absorbed when vitamin D levels are sufficient. Calcium also plays a role in how muscles contract and relax. It can be used clinically for osteoporosis, high cholesterol, and PMS. Be mindful that various forms of calcium will be absorbed and assimilated in the body differently. Some research studies support the use of microcrystalline hydroxyapatite, a form of calcium from cows that is similar to our bones that seems to be assimilated better to strengthen bones.[137]

- **Magnesium**: Magnesium is another key mineral in the body with a variety of functions including helping hundreds of biochemical reactions take place. In simplistic terms, it's required for a lot of reactions and processes to occur properly in the body. Magnesium is necessary for adequate energy production, proper cardiac and nerve cell activity, blood vessel dilation, and relaxation of muscles to prevent spasms. It also helps prevent platelets from sticking together like vitamin E. Thus, magnesium can be used therapeutically for a myriad of conditions like angina, congestive heart failure, fibromyalgia, restless leg syndrome (RLS), anxiety, and asthma.

- **Iron**: Iron plays a critical role in oxygen transport as part of hemoglobin in blood. Additionally, iron helps with energy production within cells, thyroid hormone synthesis, and dopamine production. Iron absorption is improved in combination with vitamin C. Iron may be useful medically in the treatment of anemia and infertility. Notably, iron is not generally necessary as a supplement since most people absorb sufficient amounts from foods, especially meats and vegetables. In lieu of this, unnecessary supplementation can be harmful and should only be done with guidance from a trained clinician.

- **Zinc**: This mineral is needed in our bodies for protein and DNA synthesis, proper visual and immune function, sperm production, and for healing cuts, scrapes, and burns. It also has anti-inflammatory and antioxidant capacity. Zinc may be useful for sickle cell anemia, common colds, cold sores/herpes simplex, arthritis, and taste disorders. Zinc is best taken with food to prevent nausea.

- **Iodine**: Iodine is most typically noted for its association with thyroid hormone production in the body. Interestingly, goiters can form as a result of too much or too little iodine. For this reason, blood test and potentially imaging can provide more information for proper treatment. In addition, iodine has been used clinically for fibrocystic breast changes and to improve hearing.

- **Chromium**: Chromium is a mineral that is intimately associated with insulin function. As a result, chromium helps in the regulation of blood sugar levels. Chromium may be useful for diabetes, gestational diabetes, metabolic syndrome, and polycystic ovary syndrome (PCOS).

- **Selenium**: Selenium is a mineral that serves vital roles as an antioxidant and also assists with thyroid hormone conversion. It has antiviral activity and also helps regulate immune function. It may be helpful in cancer and autoimmune conditions.

In addition to the myriad of vitamins and minerals that help our bodies function optimally, there are also other substances our bodies can produce or use to improve our health. Sometimes eating foods rich in these nutrients or taking supplements containing them can be helpful.

- **CoQ10**: This is a fat-soluble substance that is one of the body's resources for energy production. It enhances immunity and prevents some of the typical changes that occur with aging. It's particularly useful for cardiovascular and neurological health. Since statins inhibit CoQ10 production in the liver, CoQ10 should be supplemented in conjunction with statins. If you or someone you know takes statins but does not take CoQ10 also, please see a health care professional regarding the matter.
- **Alpha Lipoic Acid (ALA)**: This nutrient is a potent antioxidant that works efficiently in areas of the body primarily comprised of water as well as areas that are abundant with fats. It is an antioxidant that helps recycle other antioxidants like vitamins C and E. ALA has also been shown to be helpful in normalizing blood sugar levels.
- **Bioflavonoids**: These plant-derived nutrients are abundant and provide many of the medicinal qualities we seek from certain plants. For example, there are isoflavones in soy and red clover while anthocyanins are concentrated in blackberries and red cabbage. These nutrients have various roles, but some have anti-

inflammatory action that is particularly helpful in maintaining healthy blood vessels and others have been shown to be beneficial for cardiovascular health.

- **Probiotics**: Although it may seem strange to believe that bacteria or yeast can promote health, taking a probiotic supplement is becoming more common, particularly with the ubiquitous use of prescription antibiotics that generally kill off good gut bacteria along with the bad. Most of our health is intimately related to how efficiently the digestive system functions. For this reason, having healthy gut flora is critical and can be accomplished with probiotics. Healthy "gut bugs" can help your body defeat pathogenic invaders. They also produce vitamin K and biotin. Clinically, probiotics can be helpful for many gastrointestinal problems as well as supporting general immune function.

Finally, be mindful that the supplement industry earns billions of dollars each year as consumers become more health conscious. With this in mind, recognize that supplements are not manufactured with standard protocols and different versions of the same nutrient or supplement can yield different results primarily based on the absorptive qualities. Thus, guidance from a licensed health care professional who understands these differences can be helpful.

Eat Less Sugar and Refined Grains – Even Without Diabetes

According to the CDC, diabetes is the sixth leading cause of death in the U.S. and in many cases, particularly in diabetes mellitus type II, is preventable. Increasing statistics regarding the health consequences of diets high in sugar and refined grains support the notion that eating these types of foods on a regular basis significantly increases risks for certain conditions. One study that tracked over 75,000 women for 10 years noted that a high intake of rapidly digested and absorbed carbohydrates increases the risk of coronary heart disease (CHD) independent of associated factors like diabetes and smoking.[138]

It's vitally important to understand the connection regarding how carbohydrate intake can increase lipids. Too much glucose moving throughout the bloodstream can cause micro-tears in the walls of vasculature. In an effort to repair the damage, the liver produces more cholesterol to plug up the "breaches" in the blood vessels. This is one proposed mechanism regarding how high blood sugar and high cholesterol are related.

Now, let's address insulin's role. Simple carbohydrates found in sugary treats and most refined grain products tend to increase blood sugar very rapidly. In most people, this leads to the release of insulin from specialized beta cells in the pancreas. Initially, there is a quick spurt of insulin released to accommodate rapidly rising blood sugar. Then, the release of insulin slows down because the pancreas has to make more insulin once the initial stores are depleted as typically occurs with large, American-sized meals. The extra glucose in the blood stream is then converted to fat and stored for energy later. In type II diabetes, this whole process occurs so frequently, that the pancreas begins to produce irregular insulin that is not recognized well by cells. As a result, glucose remains elevated in the blood then gets converted to fat and stored.

Let's review. When there's high glucose and relatively low insulin or high glucose and an abnormal cell response to insulin, what happens to the extra glucose? Yes, the glucose gets converted to fat and is generally stored around the gut. You've got it now!

Recognize that carbohydrate-rich foods aren't inherently bad for you. *Excess* carbohydrates are the problem since the leftover carbohydrates are converted into fat. Take your hand and place it on your abdomen near your belly button. If your stomach tends to protrude out further than any other part of your body (with the exception of breasts in well-endowed women), it's likely that the abdominal fat you're toting around is the result of overconsumption of carbohydrates, low levels of physical activity, or other hormonal imbalances.

Carbohydrate consumption can also increase production of the neurotransmitter serotonin, which was mentioned previously regarding managing stress. Since this neurotransmitter "relieves anxiety and produces a sense of euphoria," this may explain why so many of us succumb to the pleasure of carbohydrate-rich treats on a frequent basis. Many of us are numb and oblivious regarding how much sugar and refined grains we actually eat. The Recommended Daily Allowance (RDA) for carbohydrates is 130 grams per day for adults and children. Just to put this amount into perspective, one slice of whole wheat bread contains around 12 grams of carbohydrates.[25] So, if you eat a sandwich for lunch that is 24 grams of carbohydrates, which is almost 20 percent of the amount allowed daily. If you add a bag of potato chips and a soda, this will be around 50 percent of your daily allowance. See how quickly the carbohydrates add up!

It's also important to address the *types* of carbohydrates consumed. When God originally designed the Earth and us, He set things to work in harmony with one another. This is why whole grains and fresh fruits don't tend to cause the same metabolic response in the body compared to refined grains and concentrated sugar. This is primarily because whole grains and fruit also contain fiber, which we cannot digest. Interestingly, fiber acts like a broom and a sponge simultaneously in our digestive systems by moving consumed foods through and absorbing some water along the way to prevent blockages. These qualities of fiber slow glucose absorption effectively. It is important to note when reading nutrition labels that fiber can be subtracted from the total carbohydrates listed. Thus, 2 grams of the slice of whole wheat bread that contains 12 grams of carbohydrates would only count as 10 grams of total carbohydrates since the fiber wouldn't be digested. These are the usable carbs or net carbs.[139] Additionally, fruit contains lots of water, which tends to dilute the sugars present making them less likely to spike blood sugar unless the pancreas is not functioning properly.

With advances in agriculture and mass-produced sugar utilizing new technology, our bodies are experiencing different problems from consumption of the adulterated foods. Since refined grain and sugary treats are readily available, accessible, and affordable, the healthcare industry is finally recognizing the consequences of this pervasive problem. The cohort study of women mentioned earlier in this section further concluded "the current low-fat, high carbohydrate diet recommended in the United States may not be optimal for the prevention of CHD and could actually increase the risk in individuals with high degrees of insulin resistance and glucose intolerance." Thus, there are growing concerns regarding why we should reassess what is best for our bodies even if we have not been diagnosed with diabetes.

Overcoming Carbohydrate Cravings

So how can we overcome the *habit* of eating things that both taste good and make us feel so good? Delighted you'd like to know! Actually, you already know because the Holy Spirit living in you knows all things. Since we're all unique individuals, this is definitely the best approach because what works for one person may not necessarily work for everyone else. Thus, the very first thing to do is pray about it! Be honest with yourself. Then take your concern to God humbled by your need for Him to give you the courage and strength to activate self-control, a fruit of the Spirit.

After presenting your request, once you've gotten a response from God regarding what to do, follow through diligently. If you're still waiting for a response, you can activate your faith with action.[140] Here are a few tips that may be helpful:

- *Believe* you can successfully implement the necessary dietary changes. Since you just finished praying a faithful prayer to our omnipotent Father, you can rely on Him to help you with the dietary transition and be successful.
- Next, before attempting to make changes write down everything you eat for one week. Include the amounts

too. You can just jot the info down on paper or record it on your phone. Alternatively, you may find food tracking resources like these noted here helpful.

http://www.myfooddiary.com

http://www.fitday.com

http://www.mynetdiary.com,

http://www.myfitnesspal.com

- After keeping a record of what you ate, do an analysis on the foods you consumed. Then, based on the information you've read thus far in this book, do you think most of the foods are really good, healthy choices or are they nutrient deficient and likely to lead to health problems if consumed persistently long-term? Answer this question for each food. Then determine the total percentage of the food you ate that was healthy vs. not really healthy. A good initial goal for most people is to aim for 70 percent healthy and 30 percent not really healthy. Then transition over the course of a year or two closer to a 90 percent:10 percent ratio. By leaving some flexibility in your dietary choices, you are never completely restricted from enjoying treats occasionally, and you will be more likely to adopt this method of food choice as a lifestyle, not a temporary fix.

- You may also benefit from keeping a record of any symptoms or discomfort you notice associated with certain foods or amounts of foods eaten. For example, you may feel tired after eating a sandwich with a side of potato salad. However, you may notice that if you eat the sandwich with avocado and bean chips, you feel great. These small details can help you eat foods that work well with your body.

- Take note of any habits you've developed regarding when you are most likely to indulge in foods that are not health promoting. Try to develop new ways of getting through those moments while eating healthy foods or doing different activities that are better, acceptable substitutes.

- If you're generally healthy already, choose one to two times during the week when eating one of your favorite treats is permissible. A long as the proportion of the treat or dessert is reasonable, you can have some cake! If you're not so healthy, know that eventually, you'll be able to eat some sweet treats later in moderation. In the meantime, let fruit be your dessert!

- Although this will be addressed more in the next chapter, fasting is an excellent way to reboot your taste receptors, which can help nutritious foods taste better and processed foods taste gross, i.e. extremely salty or copiously sweetened.

- Celebrate eating healthy! This will help adjust your perspective so the process of incorporating change can actually be a delightful experience for you. For example, you may select one day every week and call it "Veggie Day," "Health Promoting Day," or "Beautiful Body Day."

- Remember to be sure the thoughts you have about your health and body match with what the Bible says. Take a moment to visualize your cells becoming healthy and vibrant the way God intended them to be. Envision the blood of Jesus covering the area of your body that has been diagnosed as faulty, abnormal, or diseased and it being restored to perfect functionality. This exercise works great to annihilate worry. You don't have permission to worry.[141]

Better Protein Options

Although many health conscious people tend to adopt vegan or vegetarian diets, this may not be the best option long-term for you as an individual. In America, we generally tend to eat too much protein. As a result, livestock farmers have capitalized on ways to increase profits while decreasing costs to meet the demand for meat. For this reason, much of the beef, poultry, and fish available in most grocery stores are products from massive, livestock farming operations.

As a result of the mega-production of livestock, the nutritional value of the animal products has decreased in comparison to how most animals were raised in the past. Now, most livestock animals do not eat diets similar to what is normal for such animals. For example, under ordinary circumstances cows would primarily eat grass. However, when it was discovered that feeding cows corn increased their weight faster, man decided it was a cool idea.[142] Just as corn grain in excess fattens up humans, the same is true for cattle. Additionally, the fat ratio of the meat from a corn-fed cow differs from that of a grass-fed cow. Compounding the confusion, this corn-based diet is primarily what skews the ratio of Omega-6:Omega-3 fatty acids as discussed previously in Chapter 3. This means most of the beef available in America is an "unhealthy" option. Additionally, this is probably why beef consumption has been negatively associated with increasing rates of heart disease, diabetes, and cancer. It's fundamentally an issue regarding an imbalance of healthy fats that previously was commonplace in our diets prior to the agricultural evolution and mass processing of foods. Thus, your health outcomes may not be as significantly impacted by the fact that you like steak. Instead, your health outcomes will be more associated with the quality of the steaks you eat.

Fortunately, there are ranchers who embrace the old-fashioned way of raising cows. Products from these animals have healthy fat ratios since the cows primarily eat grass as they would normally. One study previously referenced in Chapter 3 demonstrated that the Omega-3 content in grass-fed cattle was either twice the amount or more than grain-fed cattle.[43] This improved the Omega-6:Omega-3 ratio making this type of protein source a better and healthy choice. Although it takes longer for these types of cows to gain enough weight for slaughter, the nutrient content is markedly better compared to corn or grain-fed cattle in feedlots. Not surprisingly, the Omega-6:Omega-3 ratio is true for pigs as well even though pigs tend to be the least selective regarding their diets. Interestingly, the study also highlighted attempts to alter the nutritional profile of grain-fed cattle making it more similar to that of grass-fed cattle through supplementation. For this reason, simply eating cuts of beef from grass-fed or grass-finished cattle is actually a natural, healthy source of protein.

In the same way, chickens that eat their natural diet of seeds, insects, worms, and some grain, excluding excess corn or soy, tend to produce eggs that are higher in nutrients. The meat from naturally raised chicken also has a better Omega-

6:Omega-3 ratio. The key is to recognize that "pasture fed" is the best way to identify this type of poultry. Apparently, the government allows large "confined animal feeding operations" (CAFO) to claim that the chickens are "free range." This is unfortunate since many people believe these types of eggs are a healthier option. The nutrient content in chickens and eggs from chickens that are allowed to roam about freely outside in the sunshine on pastures produce products with higher concentrated nutrients, i.e. twice as much Omega-3 fats, two-thirds more Vitamin A, three times more Vitamin E, and seven times more beta carotene.[143] Additionally, the eggs from these chickens contain one-third less cholesterol and one-quarter less saturated fat. Again, being informed about the different options for poultry products and chicken can help us make wise decisions.

Now, let's address vegetarian diets. Typically, when someone says they are vegetarian, they likely follow one of these dietary patterns while avoiding meat:

a. a well-balanced, nutrient-dense diet with a variety of vegetables and reasonable amounts of grain
b. an imbalanced, carbohydrate-rich, convenience foods based "vegetarian" diet lacking fundamental nutrients

Since most of the meat currently available in the U.S. likely has an imbalanced Omega-6:Omega-3 ratio, following a well balanced, nutrient-dense vegetarian diet definitely has its advantages. However, in order for it to be substantially advantageous, the focus of the diet must be vegetables, not grains or even fruits. By eating in this manner, one can easily consume the recommended amounts of veggies daily and have substantial amounts of antioxidants and other nutrients in their diet. One key point to be aware of regarding following a vegetarian diet though is that vegetables and fruits contain some carbohydrates. Many root vegetables like potatoes contain high amounts of carbohydrates and also should not be the focus of the diet. Since our bodies require dietary protein, beans can help fulfill this requirement. However, beans alone usually lack the complete protein profile as meat or eggs. Thus, it's important to recognize that combining legumes with certain grains can help provide complete proteins. Combinations like beans, lentils, or peanuts with rice, wheat, or corn are usually good options. There is also lots of protein packed in foods like tofu, tempeh, chia, hempseed, and quinoa (pronounced keen-wah).

Vegan diets are a bit more restrictive and pose different challenges to ensure basic nutritional needs are met. Some people choose to follow vegan diets to support and prevent mistreatment or slaughter of animals. Thus, vegans avoid consumption of all animals and also avoid consumption or use of animal products. This diet is similar to the Daniel fast short-term, which innately renders results initially due to the marked increase in consumption of nutrient dense foods such as vegetables, fruits, and grains. However, long-term effects of a vegan diet pose other concerns and may lead to negative health consequences.

Although "a vegan diet appears to be useful for increasing the intake of protective nutrients and phytochemicals and for minimizing the intake of dietary factors implicated in several chronic diseases," there are still notable nutritional deficiencies that may counter arguments in support of long-term plant-based diets.[144] For example, Omega-3 fats are most concentrated in animal products like wild-caught fish and eggs from pasture-raised chickens. Vegans and vegetarians tend to have lower blood levels of DHA and EPA, which are essential for cardiovascular health and eye and brain function. Microalgae can serve as an alternative fatty acid source for vegans. However, without EPA, taking DHA supplements alone can raise LDL cholesterol.[145]

Long-term vegan diets also compromise vitamin D levels and average about one-quarter the intake of omnivores. Since our bodies can synthesize vitamin D to an extent, some other variables may increase the likelihood of a vitamin D deficiency being more likely in vegans including darker skin, elderly people, those with limited sun exposure, and those who commonly wear sunscreen. Low vitamin D levels have been linked to increased risk of death associated with cardiovascular disease, cognitive impairment (elderly), asthma (children), and cancer.[146] Notably, supplementing with a non-animal source of vitamin D also poses a concern since vitamin D2 is not utilized as efficiently by the body as vitamin D3. Additionally, low vitamin D levels compromise bone-mineral density increasing the risks of softer bones (osteomalacia) and rickets.

Additionally, long-term vegan diets have been associated with low vitamin B12 since this vitamin is primarily found in meat or animal products. The most common initial symptom of low vitamin B12 is low energy. However, if the deficiency remains uncorrected "it can eventually cause permanent nerve damage, depression, numbness and tingling in the hands and feet, nervousness, paranoia, hyperactive reflexes, impaired memory, and behavioral changes."[147] There's additional concern for pregnant and lactating women regarding the neurological development of offspring as well. As mentioned earlier in this chapter, many of the B vitamins, particularly vitamins B-6 and B12, activate biochemical reactions in the body including the activation of enzymes. With insufficient vitamin B12, an enzyme that typically breaks down homocysteine is no longer activated so homocysteine levels typically increase. "Elevated homocysteine has been considered a risk factor for cardiovascular disease and osteoporotic bone fractures."[144] So, vegans could develop cardiovascular disease as well albeit through a different mechanism.

There are also concerns regarding possible insufficient levels of iron and zinc as a result of a vegan diet, but more research is needed to determine if naturally occurring compensatory mechanisms are sufficient. One compensatory mechanism is due to more efficient absorption of iron when coupled with vitamin C, which would be relatively abundant in a well balanced, nutrient dense vegan diet. There are also immunological responses adapted to a lower intake of zinc that may make up for lower levels of the nutrient.

There is also debate about other potential consequences due to a long-term vegan diet, including menstrual changes or complete loss of menstruation in women and balding or lower sperm counts in men. Considering fertility and hair aren't required for an individual's survival, it seems reasonable that these areas of the body would be impacted in individuals with long-term nutritionally deficient diets.

Finally, in a similar manner as the vegetarian diet, consumption of too many carbohydrates may not be healthy for an individual based on their metabolism. Thus, eating a vegan diet heavily focused on carbohydrates may not be the wisest decision in an effort to optimize health. Conducting your own thorough research coupled with speaking with your doctor about adopting a vegan diet would be ideal.

Fat Fallacy

There's a lot of misinformation regarding the "dangers of fats." Fats are not innately bad. However, it is important to recognize that the *types* of fats and the manner the fats are prepared ultimately will determine if your body will have good levels of fats. Most people don't realize how important fats are in the human body. Remember fats make up approximately 25 percent of our bodies. Fats form a protective barrier around every cell. Fats also help the nervous system, including your brain, and the immune system to function better. Fats are used to make vitamin D, hormones like estrogen and testosterone, and molecular messengers called prostaglandins. Additionally, there's even fat in your hair! For these reasons, and many others not mentioned, it is imperative that we consume healthy sources of fat since they literally become incorporated within our bodies and determine how efficiently our bodies function based on the quality of "fuel" available.

Do you recall from Chapter 3 that most of the cholesterol in your body is produced by your liver?[25,148] Although we've been conditioned to think that it only comes from dietary sources, the body actually manufactures cholesterol in response to its concentration within cells. The body also adjusts how much cholesterol is produced based on levels of ATP, an energy molecule, and insulin levels. When there's less of each, cholesterol synthesis ceases.[22] This is partly why people with insulin resistance, where insulin levels tend to be higher, often have elevated cholesterol as well.

Cholesterol serves many important roles in the body. It is a precursor to the formation of the hormones testosterone and estrogen. This is why many people who are prescribed medication to decrease their cholesterol levels may eventually have a low libido. Cholesterol also helps every cell membrane in our bodies to remain flexible and fluid like ocean waves allowing good things in and discriminating against harmful substances.

Apparently, cholesterol got such a "bad wrap" based on research endeavors from scientists like Rudolph Virchow, Ancel Keys, and others participating in the Framingham study that led to erroneous beliefs heralded by the medical community that are still widely accepted today.[149] Despite new cutting edge technology and a myriad of more research that negates the idea that elevated cholesterol levels alone increase risks of cardiovascular disease (CVD), most Americans have been conditioned to believe this is true. As a result, "low-fat," "fat-free," and "cholesterol free" food products are widely available and are considered healthier choices among consumers although many of these low-fat foods have higher amounts of sugar in them so the food tastes better. Unfortunately, after eating sugary, fat-free treats, our brains still feel that there is something more desired, probably fat. So when we eat more, our blood sugar rises as well as insulin and in turn our cholesterol levels and weight increase too. This is the reason there is a clearly defined association of CVD in patients diagnosed with diabetes, insulin resistance, and metabolic syndrome. As mentioned previously, in this subset of the population elevated levels of glucose actually contribute to damaging the intraepithelial layer of cells lining blood vessels. In response to the damage, repair mechanisms are triggered that lead to the accumulation of cells and cholesterol to patch up the damage. Thus, cholesterol isn't the real culprit. The extra sugar is. It's actually more prudent to consider mechanisms that damage the inner lining of blood vessels that lead to the cascade of events associated with cardiovascular disease than to assume dietary cholesterol is the problem.

The lifelong work of university research scientist Fred Kummerow may provide more insight about the main reasons cardiovascular disease is so common now. His findings deemed "fried foods, powdered egg yolks, excess vegetable oils, partially hydrogenated vegetable oils, and cigarette smoke as the greatest culprits in heart disease."[150] Apparently, oxysterols, found in fried foods and powdered food substances change the biochemistry of phospholipids, the molecules that make up the vast majority of the membranes surrounding cells. He found increased calcium deposits resulted from consumption of such foods. Interestingly, he also found excess consumption of vegetable oils caused the same result. He further concluded that cigarette smoke and partially hydrogenated oils interfere with proper fat metabolism interrupting blood flow, the mainstay of the end result in CVD.[149]

In another study, Kummerow looked further into how oxidation played a role in CVD. Oxidation is a simple process involving the loss of electrons, small negatively charged particles in atoms, which occurs in both living organisms as well as in the environment. As simple as the process seems, products that are oxidized can cause damage to the surroundings if antioxidant levels are insufficient. When fats are oxidized, they form free radicals that actively attempt to regain the lost electrons. The fats may transform into other variations of free radicals since they are extremely unstable. Then, eventually they form lipid peroxides. Kummerow's research team found higher levels of oxidation products (LPX, or lipid peroxides) in patients who had cardiac catheters recently placed. The cholesterol levels of the same patients were analyzed as well and the researchers found no correlation.[151] Another noteworthy point also addressed from this research was that age was not a factor in the findings. So if you're older, this doesn't necessarily increase your risks of CVD. Instead, increased oxidation of fats combined with low antioxidant status increases risks of CVD significantly.

Another factor that has recently gained the attention of researchers and well-informed health care practitioners, relates to the sub-types of cholesterol. You may not know this based on a standard lipid panel, but there are different types of LDL and HDL. The variations are based on proteins imbedded within LDL and HDL, which are essentially spherical shuttles that transport cholesterol throughout the body. Interestingly, knowing the levels of each subtype can more accurately determine if there is a greater chance of a person being at risk for CVD. In addition, treatment approaches can be more precise and effective. For this reason, it's important to work with health care providers who understand how to comprehensively address elevated lipids instead of initially prescribing medication that may or may not be effective. Another noteworthy point regarding the blood tests that can further extrapolate which types of cholesterol are elevated is that there may be a genetic component called lipoprotein A, Lp(a), that could significantly increase risks of CVD in people who may not even have elevated cholesterol. Again, it's imperative to work with health care providers who know when this may be an important consideration based on your individual medical history.

Triglycerides, also known as triacylglycerols (TAGs), are another type of fat the body produces to use for energy later if needed. Do you remember that carbohydrates can be used to make fat in the body? This is where the process occurs biochemically. In short, a bunch of molecules and enzymes work together inside cells to assemble triglycerides, which are composed of a glycerol molecule at the head and three fatty acid tails attached. Take note that this is where the essential fatty acids, Omega-3 and Omega-6, are incorporated and stored. When necessary, fatty acids are freed to provide energy in many tissues throughout the body, especially in the liver and muscles. Additionally, fatty acids are used for the tails on the phospholipids that make up the majority of the cell membrane as mentioned previously. It's important to recognize that two different situations in cells can trigger triglyceride synthesis. First, glucose can be used in the liver and in fat cells to make the glycerol head of triglycerides. There's also a second way the liver produces the initial glycerol used in production of triglycerides by using a special enzyme. So, putting all this fancy biochemical information together leads to one major point: "when plasma glucose (and insulin) levels are low, there's limited availability for production of triglycerides."[22] Again, keeping blood sugar levels in a healthy range can prevent elevated triglyceride levels.

Healthy Fats

The right types of fats have anti-inflammatory properties and usually have moderate amounts of Omega-6 fatty acids and higher levels of Omega-3 fatty acids. Foods that contain cholesterol can be good for your health since cholesterol is used to create products that support cellular function and improve your immune system, mood, and libido. Excluding cholesterol from your diet is not necessary because your liver makes most of the cholesterol in your body anyway. As with all things, avoid going overboard though!

If you happen to have been diagnosed with high cholesterol, or hypercholesterolemia, there are other concerns that should be addressed by your health care provider. In particular, if you have been prescribed a statin for treatment, but your lipid levels have not improved, it's possibly because the mechanism statins use to decrease cholesterol is not addressing the source of the problem in your body. Statins simply block a liver enzyme called HMG Co-A reductase. This enzyme promotes the production of cholesterol, which is necessary for "fluid" cell membranes and sufficient hormone levels. In addition, other biochemical processes that rely on this enzyme are impeded hence the reason CoQ10 must be supplemented while on statin therapy as mentioned previously. Because of misinformation, widely accepted fallacies about cholesterol levels in research, and increased pharmaceutical profits with the continued use of statins, the root of the problem remains unaddressed and cardiovascular disease remains the leading cause of death in the U.S. It's time to start asking your physician direct questions if your health isn't improving so you won't be a statistic based on how current systems manage the health of millions of Americans.

The fats your body needs and can metabolize effectively are present in animal products from grass-fed cows, pasture-raised chickens, and wild fish. (Note: Some goat and sheep producers feed grains to the animals instead of allowing them to freely consume their natural diet.[152] Thus it's wise to verify what the animals consumed.) Also, pork may be an option as well if the rancher closely monitored their diets and gave the pigs a healthier diet rich in vegetables and healthy fats.

There are also healthy fats in a myriad of vegetable oils although many naturally contain higher amounts of Omega-6 fats. For this reason, it may be best to consume these types of oils in moderation and focus more on those with higher Omega-3 content like flaxseed, walnut, and peanut oils. Be mindful that most oils are quite sensitive to heat and can transform into trans-fats simply by a change in orientation in relation to a double bond. Thus, using unheated oil is likely the best option. Generally, low heat, less than 320°F, is acceptable for use with most oils like extra virgin olive oil, walnut oil, and hempseed oil. Moderate heat, less than 400°F, is acceptable when using macadamia nut oil and grapeseed oil.

Interestingly, coconut oil should also be a consideration. Although this oil is rich in saturated fat, most of this fat is medium-chained lauric acid, which is easily absorbed and metabolized (just like the medium-chain fat in breast milk). It doesn't negatively affect lipid levels. In addition, coconut oil boasts of added benefits uniquely possessing antibacterial and antiviral action.[153] With a smoke point around 350°F, this should also be considered when heating. Finally, avocado oil is essentially the "big guns" for heating oil without denaturing it or changing it into trans-fat. Avocado oil has a smoke point just over 500°C and also has high amounts of vitamin E.[154] Take note that many oils used in packaged products are not considered healthy options namely canola, corn, and soy oils since most are likely GMO in the U.S. Since we're unsure of the outcome of consumption of GMO products (especially in concentrated forms like oils), let's just avoid them collectively and see what happens!

Water

Since approximately 50 to 70 percent of the human body is water, it makes sense that water is an essential consideration for optimizing health. Water is required for and produced from many biochemical reactions in the body. It also helps clear wastes and toxic matter out of the body. For this reason, drinking sufficient water daily is essential for optimal health. One common suggestion is to drink at least half of your body weight in ounces. However, this may be too general in some instances so adjusting water intake based on specific factors seems more reasonable. For example, living in areas where humidity is often low or temperatures are excessively hot or cold typically increases basic needs for water. Exercise or extended periods of exertion also increase the need for water. On the contrary, less water may be necessary for people who are fasting or for those who require dialysis.

Other reasons to increase or decrease water intake may exist based on your unique circumstance. Thus, it's best to discuss something as simple as water intake with your doctor. If it doesn't seem important to your doctor, gently remind him or her that most of the body *is* water so it should be addressed.

There are numerous companies that purify water and sell it to the general public since most water treatment facilities have less stringent standards for water purification. This is probably why some grocery stores allot nearly half of an aisle to stocking different types of water! Additionally, there are some companies that offer water filtration systems for homes and businesses further complicating the decision process. As a result, simply choosing what type of water to drink can be challenging.

Consider the basic structure of water—two hydrogen atoms and an oxygen atom bonded together. That's it! Nothing else is chemically needed or required for the molecule to be water. So, if there were a preferred type of water to drink, distilled water would be best. Some of us may recall the distillation process from chemistry class. A liquid containing water is heated and upon reaching 100°C (or 212°F), the water in the solution begins to boil and then evaporates from the mixture. Fancy glassware is then used to contain and redirect the steam, which is pure water. As the steam cools, it condenses and is collected in a separate container. Unfortunately, production of distilled water is quite costly because of the energy output necessary to heat large amounts of water. Additionally, distillation probably isn't the most sustainable mechanism for water purification. Since it is just water, some people believe this increases the chance that essential minerals may be flushed from the body as a result of the varied concentrations of the distilled water and other solutes required by the body.

Water purified through reverse osmosis presents another alternative that is not as costly as distillation since pressure is used to filter the water. The process involves high pressure being used to push water across membranes to filter the water. Interestingly, the pressure is so great, that once the water is filtered, the energy moving the water can be used to create more pressure to repeat the process making reverse osmosis an energetically efficient process.[155] Like distillation, reverse osmosis removes essentially everything out of the water including "pharmaceutical and industrial waste, heavy metals, chemicals, radioactive particles, fluoride, and chlorine."[156] Unfortunately, it also removes many trace minerals from the water and may deplete minerals from the body when consumed regularly.

In lieu of the depletion of minerals from distillation and reverse osmosis, a simple solution is to add minerals back into the water prior to consumption. Since this typically isn't done following the distillation process, you may need to add them yourself by using concentrated mineral drops. Another mechanism to replenish minerals is by seasoning foods with Celtic or Himalayan sea salt, which are naturally high in minerals and are preferred forms of salt in comparison to typical table salt that tends to be devoid of trace minerals.

Lastly, alkaline water has a higher pH than pure water and is promoted as a better option for health since many infectious processes and cancer tend to falter in alkaline environments. The pH of a liquid is a numerical method of quantifying the concentrations of hydrogen (H^+) or hydroxide (OH^-) ions in substances. Acidic solutions have more H^+ ions while alkaline or basic substances tend to have more OH^- ions.) Mass production and supply of alkaline water may have originated from the idea that spring water is naturally slightly alkaline due to trace minerals. Choosing alkaline water should be based on personal preference. However, if your diet contains sufficient vegetables for a sustained period of time, the fluid around your cells will naturally be alkaline. As a result, slightly increasing your pH by drinking alkaline water wouldn't be necessary. At the same time, alkaline water can neutralize stomach acid, which could negatively impede digestion, especially for protein assimilation and activation of other gastrointestinal processes that are stimulated by low pH.[157] For this reason, if drinking alkaline water seems like an ideal option for you, it may be wise to consider drinking it between meals. A quick, cost effective solution that surprisingly has an alkalizing effect in the body is drinking water with freshly squeezed lemon juice. Although lemon juice is acidic, in our bodies, it helps fluids to be slightly alkaline. Notably, pre-squeezed lemon juice is not ideal for such use and may be deficient in antioxidants compared to fresh lemon juice. Another option is to obtain fresh spring water, which may be available in your area. (Visit www.findaspring.com for more information.)

Regardless of the type of water you choose, be sure to drink enough so that your urine is light-yellow and avoid drinking water that has been stored in plastic bottles for an extended period of time—years or longer. Particular caution is advisable when it's possible that the water bottle has been heated during storage or left in a hot car. Research suggests that toxins in the plastic may seep into the water making it harmful.[158] (This is an even greater concern when the contents stored in plastic bottles contain fat.) Thus, a better solution is to opt for refillable sources of water, which also decreases wastes in the environment. Look for water bottles that have numbers 2, 4 or 5 on the bottom of the bottle in the center of the arrows shaped in a triangle. These types of plastic don't contain some of the more deleterious compounds that affect hormones.

Rotational & Seasonal Diets

Have you ever noticed how some fruits and vegetables aren't readily available at some times throughout the year? For example, you'd be hard pressed to find fresh, ripe strawberries in December or a pumpkin in April. As Ecclesiastes 3:1 reminds us, every thing has a season. This includes fruits and vegetables coming into harvest. In lieu of this, it may be reasonable to infer that our bodies may fair best on the foods that are actually in season versus the overpriced, nutrient deficient and shipped from far away varieties of fruits and vegetables that tend to persist in supermarkets throughout the year.

There are a few reasons to consider eating foods that grow in-season. Once produce is harvested, nutrient levels begin declining. The rate of this decline depends on several environmental factors like ambient temperature and humidity as well as the type of produce itself. In lieu of this, it makes sense to attempt to consume produce as soon as possible closer to the time it was harvested. Additionally, recently harvested foods tend to taste better since they are fresher.

Another advantage from consuming produce in season is

that this type of consumption is sustainable.[159] It's the way things were supposed to happen as originally designed by God. It is also much easier to cultivate produce during the season that is most conducive for growth. Some seeds and plants need variable temperatures during the dormant stage of growth either when all the action is happening under the soil or when the tree appears barren. By allowing ample time for the plants to go through the necessary growth phases, the process of producing a harvest is simplified.

As mentioned previously, food that's harvested in season, can come from local farms and decrease the necessity of transport. Many advocates who support purchasing local foods do so to decrease the impact on the environment from transporting food. This helps decrease use of fuel and associated pollution.

Another reason to eat in season that may not be as noticeable is what happens inside our bodies when we eat the same foods year round. Interestingly, food sensitivities, a milder form of allergic responses, are becoming more common perhaps as a result of homogeneous diets. Thus, if you generally consume a limited number of foods (about 50) year round without pausing for intermittent periods or expanding the variety at some points, you could be triggering a subclinical immune reaction to these foods. When this happens, your gastrointestinal system loses its ability to absorb nutrients properly and your immune system begins attacking proteins from the food. When nutrient absorption decreases coupled with a distracted immune system response, a myriad of symptoms can result. Many times unhealthy skin reflects this underlying problem. However, it's also common for people to experience digestive issues, unclear thinking or fatigue and food cravings due to food sensitivities as well.[160] In lieu of this, it's important to eat based on the saying that "variety is the spice of life."

Depending on where you live, produce may come into harvest at variable times during the year throughout the United States. A wonderful reference to help you determine which foods are in season in your area is www.pickyourown.org. On this website, you can select your state to determine when common produce is harvested. By following this list, you can choose the fruits and veggies that are readily available in your area. The cost should also be notably cheaper in comparison to other produce transported from elsewhere.

Exercise

Exercise is one of the best strategies for optimal health! It helps to rapidly circulate blood throughout your body particularly during cardiovascular exercise or other activities that increase your heart rate. This results in improved oxygenation of cells, improved metabolism, more effective immune function, and better nutrient distribution throughout your body.

For weight loss, working out on an empty stomach when you initially wake up in the morning is advantageous. At this time, your body has rested and regenerated. Also, hormonally, your cortisol levels should be highest at this time of day which can help you power through the workout. Some studies suggest that more growth hormone is secreted when you practice high intensity interval workouts (HIIT).[161] This is valuable info since growth hormone is associated with increased fat burning and muscle growth.

Incorporating weight-bearing exercise into your regimen is wise since muscle burns fat. Once you've strengthened your muscles, you can just sit around while extra calories are burned off ... well, as long as you're not munching on unhealthy snacks while sitting around!

Although the physical benefits of exercise should be sufficient enough to motivate many people to begin incorporating some form of exercise in their routine, there are also mental health benefits as well. Regular exercise lifts a depressed mood having an "antidepressant-like" effect without unwanted side effects. It also has been noted to improve brain function as well![162] So if you want to be smart and happy, this is an ideal reason to put forth more effort to go to the gym or even just workout at home.

Since we're all getting older, remember that movement is the No. 1 way to prevent many of the physical ailments of the elderly. Maintaining flexibility and keeping muscles strong are definite keys to optimize your health.

Finally, don't deceive yourself if you're thin! If you don't work out regularly, you're out of shape. Being svelte does not automatically suggest that you are healthy. Recognize that although obesity does increase the risks of certain health problems, these health problems may also be issues for adults with normal body weights who are inactive. Thus, you must be proactive and exercise too, even if your goal is not weight loss.

For your convenience, here are some strategies to help you work out regularly:

- o   Add it to your schedule (now)! Since we're all so busy these days, everything that must get done should be planned ahead of time. Incorporating exercise into your schedule should not be an exception. Pause reading for a brief moment and set a reminder on your preferred electronic device to prompt you to work out. Set the reminder to repeat until you've established the habit.

o Ask a friend to join you or to hold you accountable. Some of us are more likely to thrive at certain tasks when we have to be accountable to someone. If accountability helps you fulfill commitments, don't waste time trying to be consistent on your own. Enlist help by selecting a good friend or coach to help you reach your goals.

o Start working out for short increments of time. Then, increase the amount of time as you get accustomed to it. I usually ask patients if they can work out for 15 minutes. Usually, this isn't a problem. Once they've incorporated working out for 15 minutes three to five days a week into their schedule, it is easier to increase the amount of time spent working out. Often, the duration and intensity of the workouts increase as benefits are observed. Additionally, it's best for inactive people to take it slowly with their initial workouts to prevent injury and to get their bodies accustomed to exertion. Of course, seek the counsel of a health care professional before starting any new exercise regimen.

It may also be helpful to include a reward system for yourself based on how frequently you maintain your workout schedule. Of course, edible rewards may be counterproductive so aim to buy yourself a new outfit since your old clothes will be too baggy anyway! Alternatively, you can book an appointment at a local spa or go to a local sport event. Just do something to keep yourself motivated so it feels like you've earned a reward for a job well done.

~

In summary, in order to ultimately optimize your health and significantly decrease the chances of developing a chronic disease, discuss these ideas with your doctor. Hopefully, they will support and encourage you to take steps toward achieving optimal health. Additionally, if you have been taking prescription medications, you should meet with your doctor before implementing new strategies so you can work together to accomplish your long-term health goals safely. There are numerous recipes available on the Internet and in cookbooks that can help simplify this process. So go in faith informed and ready to experience your healthiest self!

Chapter Six: The "F" Word

Fortunately, this isn't a book where profane words pop up so you can relax! However, there is an F-word mentioned throughout the Bible that when practiced can significantly improve your relationship with God and simultaneously impact health. This word is *fasting*.

Because fasting can be quite uncomfortable during the first couple of days, people typically stray away from trying it. In general, many people in the U.S. have an antagonistic view to this spiritual practice that doubles as an ancient practice for spiritual enlightenment and purification. Additionally, many medical providers generally don't recommend fasting for patients unless the patient is temporarily preparing for a procedure or imaging. Sometimes fasting may also be suggested if negative medication interactions are likely when taken with food. Thus, therapeutic fasting for both spiritual and physical reasons has not generally been embraced. Hopefully, this chapter will enlighten you regarding many of the positive benefits of fasting.

Physical Effects and Benefits of Fasting

During fasting, numerous metabolic processes that typically occur during the "well-fed" state cease. The body transitions from storing consumed food in the form of glycogen, fat, and protein to breaking down the stored sources for fuel. Thus, the body begins breakdown processes and uses what's already available to help cells throughout the body function to sustain life.

The initial source of depleted fuel is glycogen, which is stored in the liver and in muscles. Glycogen is comprised of numerous glucose molecules connected together that can quickly be separated so free glucose molecules are available to enter and energize cells. This storage form of glucose is our main source of fuel once glucose levels in our blood decline an hour or so following our last meal. Thus, when we haven't eaten for a few hours, glycogen breakdown begins to prevent rapid drops in our blood sugar.

Rapid declines in blood sugar can be uncomfortable because they can lead to dizziness, shaking, nausea, or irritability. This is why the initial phases of fasting can be difficult for some people. Glycogen release serves as a buffer for our bodies to prevent rapid blood sugar declines from occurring as long as we eat in regular intervals. Notably, glycogen is nearly depleted from the liver after only about 10 to 18 hours.[22] This is one reason eating breakfast is so important. It helps prompt our metabolic rate to rev back up and stops our bodies from transitioning into the conservation mode adopted in the early stages of fasting. The liver also can make glucose through a process called gluconeogenesis, which requires products from fat breakdown.

Fasting that continues beyond glycogen depletion forces the body to find other sources of energy. Typically this process takes about three days of water fasting in order for the process to kick into full gear. Stored fat is a good option for fuel since it can be used to help the liver make a bit more glucose through gluconeogenesis. Fat can also be used to produce ketones, which can be used to sustain energy and proper organ function, especially in the brain, during fasting. Ketones are small molecules detectable in urine and blood that can be used by cells to make energy and sustain life during extended periods when food is not consumed. However, this process is not as efficient as the typical metabolism of glucose.

During periods of food avoidance, the body no longer has to exert energy metabolizing food so this is an ideal time for "body-cleansing" to take place. Since 70 to 80 percent of our immune system is located in and around the gastrointestinal system, the body can focus on other areas and effectively expunge things that should not be in cells that generally are not prioritized. When fasting, immune cells go on excursions throughout the body playing "which one of these is not like the other?" Once foreign substances, toxic molecules, or abnormal cells or structures are discovered, they are destroyed and banished from the body. While fasting, many toxins and waste products are mobilized, or are liberated, from fat, which harbors many of the toxins in our bodies. Over time, fasting results in decreased "body-burden" which helps people feel better. This is likely why recent health fads have focused on "detoxification." Although our bodies possess mechanisms of clearing out wastes, fasting provides an opportunity for more profound, deeper cleansing.

Many types of medical conditions can potentially be alleviated and sometimes even cured simply by fasting. These conditions include allergies, autoimmune diseases, cancer, skin and digestive problems, obesity, chronic infections, and arthritis.[26] Although fasting is a great option that only requires intention and the temporary "slaughter" of one's will, it is not advisable to fast for extended periods of time without medical supervision, especially for people previously diagnosed with chronic diseases or who take certain medications. Fortunately, there are medical professionals and centers that offer this particular service. (See the appendix for a few resources.)

Why Should We Fast in a Spiritual Sense?

Although it seems fasting is not practiced as often as it was during biblical times, fasting still has spiritual benefits as well. During a fast, there's a unique opportunity to cease from the typical demands of life to experience moments of peace, stillness, and serenity that generally aren't as easily obtainable during our typical schedules. During a fast, we position ourselves humbly before God and depend on His Word for nourishment. This makes hearing His still, soft voice easier.

When we make a decision to fast in order to get direction from God regarding a specific matter, especially amongst a group of believers, this is a *proclaimed fast* according to Kenneth Copeland.[163] The book of Esther highlights just how powerful and effective fasting and prayer can be when we need direction from the Lord. The biblical account describes how Esther was chosen to be queen and was challenged to use her position of authority to save the Jews, her own people.[164] In summary, one of the king's honored royal officials, Haman, deliberately established a law to destroy, kill, and annihilate the Jews.[165] When Mordecai, Esther's uncle, heard of the plan, he attempted to gain the attention of the queen to take a stand for her people and charged her that she had "come to her royal position for such a time as this."[166] At this point, Esther established a proclaimed fast amongst herself, her attendants, and all the Jews. During this time, they fasted and prayed. Esther sought God's direction regarding what she needed to do to prevent the annihilation of her people. Once the three-day fast was over, Esther went to the king and invited him to multiple celebrations held in his honor so he would be more receptive toward her. The king loved her so much that he was willing to give her up to half of his kingdom! Led by God, Esther recognized the most opportune time to make her request. As a result, Esther was able to make a few political decisions allowing the Jews an opportunity to defend themselves, and God helped her to deliver the Jews. During the battle, 10 of Haman's sons were killed and later, Haman was hung on the gallows that he'd originally created for Mordecai's execution. God helped direct and orchestrate this outcome. The fast helped establish "unity and singleness of purpose" resulting in God's will ultimately being done.[163]

We can also endeavor to do a *personal fast*. This type of fast is a personal decision that we do privately as an individual to hear God clearly or seek His guidance on a personal matter. This is the type of fast Jesus did for 40 days and nights when He was led by the Holy Spirit into the desert to be tempted by Satan.[167] Personal fasting won't earn you any "brownie points" with God. Our willful act of self-denial via fasting most certainly cannot move the hand of God based on our sacrifice. However, through a personal fast, we put ourselves in a position of humility, which changes us from the inside making our hearts more malleable for God's use. Jesus promised when we do such fasts, God will see it and reward us openly.[168]

Fasting can help you accomplish other things as well. Fasting helps strengthen your spirit so that your flesh can't sway you as easily. The regular practice of fasting can help us successfully do what Paul charged us to do in Galatians 5:16 and "live by the Spirit." This is particularly helpful regarding eating foods that we know are not healthy for us. Your flesh is the part of you that craves sweet treats, fried foods, and other deceptive delights. Fasting can provide "deliverance from evil spirits and (these) addictive habits."[169] The Holy Spirit living in you wants you to eat healthy, whole foods and take care of the temple that God loaned you. Conveniently, fasting resets your taste buds making eating healthy foods significantly easier after a fast. Be mindful though that reintroduction of foods high in sugar or salt after a fast can also quickly stimulate your taste buds to continue having a preference for sugary and salty treats.

Fasting also strengthens your spirit. As a believer with the Holy Spirit living in you, your spirit is connected to God based on His triune nature. Since we can't operate in the flesh and the spirit simultaneously as the natures are diametrically opposed to one another, we "feed" and strengthen one while weakening the other. Fasting feeds the spirit man, because we are no longer attending to the normal urge or sensation to eat. As a result, the spirit man is better able to dictate how the body operates—in the Spirit or the flesh.

The spiritual benefits from fasting can be summarized as follows: It helps us draw close to God and get guidance if needed, overcome the flesh, humble ourselves, and obtain spiritual breakthroughs.[170] With this in mind coupled with the myriad of physical benefits, Christians should strongly consider implementing fasting regularly. Although the initial transition may not feel so pleasant, long-term benefits are worth the temporary sacrifice.

Types of Fasts

There are a few different types of fasts that can offer both spiritual and physical opportunities for purging. If you endeavor to try fasting, be sure to get clearance from your physician first. Safe fasting is the goal and various phases of fasting present different metabolic challenges. Be mindful that if the physician you are attempting to get clearance from has never fasted before or assisted other patients with fasting, it would be wise to seek another opinion due to much skepticism regarding fasting in mainstream medicine. With proper medical guidance, fasting can be a bit easier on the body and more effective when detoxification support is provided either before or during the fast if possible. Be aware that good options are available if you choose to fast.

The Daniel Fast:

The Daniel fast, in a general sense, is a vegetarian diet that primarily includes fruits, vegetables, and whole grains. Nuts, seeds, high quality oils, seasonings, and water, of course, are also permissible during this type of fast. .[171] It is typically done for 21 consecutive days. This type of fast restricts the "pleasurable" foods we may have grown accustomed to.[172] Although food is consumed during this particular fast, it is still beneficial since it incorporates foods that are generally easy for most people to digest and assimilate. In addition, nutrition intake is boosted for most people adapting this type of fast because more vegetables and fruits are consumed.

If you plan to do the Daniel fast, it may also be wise to consider eliminating your own food sensitivities. By doing so, your immune system can more effectively carry out body cleansing and detoxification, even while you're eating! There are specific lab tests that can be ordered by a naturopathic physician or holistic health care practitioner to determine if you have any food sensitivities.

Partial Fast:
Partial fasting is essentially like the Daniel fast in that the person doing the fast can still eat. However, the particular foods avoided during a partial fast can be highly variable. For example, one may endeavor to go on a partial fast by consuming 100 percent vegetables for a certain period of time while avoiding all other foods. Alternatively, another person may adapt a partial fast by giving up their most beloved food for a certain period of time, such as no potato chips for three months. Although this type of fasting can be quite variable, it still can provide added health benefits based on the extent, type, and quality of foods avoided or incorporated.

Intermittent Fast:
Intermittent fasting involves refraining from eating for a specified amount of time then returning to eating food as before. Usually, this type of fasting is only done over short periods of time lasting about 18 to 24 hours each week. Interestingly, this type of fasting has been well researched and much of the data supports the idea that restraining from food consumption and decreasing overall caloric intake for short

periods can result in significant health benefits including, but not limited to, lower cholesterol and blood pressure, fewer degenerative diseases, and weight loss.[173]

Since this type of fasting doesn't require any changes to your current food preparation plan, intermittent fasting is easily adaptable. It saves time and money as a result. Easing into food abstention can be challenging for some people. Thus, if you are interested in this type of fast, it's best to determine the time of day you are typically most hungry and eat a good healthy meal at that time. Then, avoid eating again until after 18 to 24 hours. Based on the duration of the fasting interval, it would be wise to start eating again with a small light meal to initially reintroduce food. Then allow yourself to eat again a few hours later if you're hungry.

Juice Fast:
Drinking fresh juices for a specified period of time is generally considered a form of fasting also. Most people who engage in this type of fasting actually feel like they are fasting since no food is consumed with this type of fast. Actually though, this is medically considered a type of elimination diet, where foods that may trigger inflammation or an unnecessary immune response are eliminated from the diet temporarily to provide some degree of therapeutic relief.[174] This type of fasting offers more profound detoxification effects as caloric restriction is pronounced on a liquid diet and with the gastrointestinal system only required to attend to assimilation of liquids, digestive processes are easy so more cleaning can occur in other parts of the body. However, it is important to note that fruit juice naturally contains high amounts of sugar, and it's

135

best to consume diluted fruit juices when fasting, i.e. 50 percent juice and 50 percent water. So if you'd like to try fruit juice, mix about the same amount of water to it before drinking it. Vegetable juices from carrots, beets or other root vegetables likely contain high amounts of sugar and are also best diluted. Also, adding lemon or apple juice to a vegetable juice blend can improve the taste of juice especially from green leafy vegetables.

Notably, it's not ideal to attempt a juice fast using many of the juice options available in grocery stores since they usually contain high fructose corn syrup or other additives that would be counterproductive during a fast. Freshly made juice from whole fruit is best. It can be frozen and consumed later if necessary.

Since juice is concentrated, it's also very important to use organic fruits and vegetables during a juice fast. Otherwise, you'll be drinking concentrated pesticide residues and undermining the entire process. If organic fruits and vegetables are not accessible, peeling the food prior to juicing can be an alternative. However, this can significantly decrease the nutrient content obtained from the juice. So again, the best option is to use organic whole fruits and vegetables.

Water Fast:
Technically, this is most profound way to fast since consumption is completely avoided with the exception of drinking water. The other types of "fasts" mentioned can help, but physiologically water fasting is the most efficient for the body. Christians are particularly familiar with this type of fast since Jesus was led by the Holy Spirit into the desert and water

fasted for 40 days. Water fasting allows the most profound degree of detoxification and is also the most risky and uncomfortable for most people. It's particularly tricky for people taking prescription medications to participate in this type of fast because medications are often supposed to be taken with food. If this is your situation, remain faithful about this being an option for you. It is possible for most people to water fast with proper medical supervision. The length or duration of the water fast may need to be incrementally increased as your body adapts to deeper levels of detoxification.

Dry Fasting:
This type of fasting is not advisable since it involves no eating or drinking, not even water! Since our bodies are primarily made of water and since the fluids circulating in our body assist with the excretion of wastes, avoiding drinking water during fasting could be detrimental. This type of fasting is not prudent. During water fasting, the desire for water may actually decrease somewhat, but eventually you will be thirsty. When this happens, drink up!

Chapter Seven: Your Prosperous Health Plan

Do you think God intended for us to be sick or live healthy, whole, and meaningful lives? Do you believe He wants us to suffer pain or to be free from both physical and emotional pain? Do you embrace the idea that sickness and infirmity are simply part of our human existence now but everything will be perfect once we get to heaven? Interestingly, we may have various perspectives and opinions about what our health should be like. However, God made it very clear what His original intention was regarding sickness and disease.

In Isaiah, the promise of Jesus' coming, punishment, and death addressed how we have been healed. "But He was wounded for our transgressions, He was bruised for our guilt *and* iniquities; the chastisement [needful to obtain] peace *and* well-being for us was upon Him, and with the stripes [that wounded] Him we are healed *and* made whole."[175] Transgressions are defined as acts that violate or go against a law or rule. Chastisement is immoral or grossly unfair behavior. To put this all together, essentially, Jesus took on the punishment for our sin and sickness. It wasn't fair for Him to be treated this way since He was without sin. First Peter 2 further expounds upon God's word being fulfilled. "He personally bore our sins in His [own] body on the tree [as on an altar and offered Himself on it], that we might die (cease to exist) to sin and live to righteousness. By His wounds you have been healed."[176] So it's already been done! It's already complete through Jesus! The issue most Christians have though is knowing how to connect to the supernatural healing power that's available through faith and trusting God's Word.

Sin & Sickness

Sickness is not from God. Sickness occurs as a result of sin.[177,178] The sin resulting in sickness may or may not be related to your personal sins or even the sins of your parents or grandparents. Regardless of the source, since sin is the default mechanism here on earth, sickness came along with it. Sin and sickness come from the same source, the devil. Thus, it is important for Christians to recognize the true source of the problem. It's time for us to stop allowing and passively permitting the devil to deceive us into thinking we have absolutely no power, authority, or control over what happens to us, particularly regarding our health. This is deception that we must dare to challenge. The healing ministry of the church did not stop with the advent of pharmaceutical medications! Let's use God's Word and His promises to overcome sin and sickness.

Why You Have Not Been Healed

Believing what modern medicine says about your condition may be one of the primary reasons it has been difficult for you to be healed. Many TV programs and commercials make it seem as if health problems are incurable and the only solution or option for relief of symptoms is through the use of medications. Of course, there are times when symptom relief could be lifesaving and is thus quite appropriate. However, many mainstream treatments simply temporarily stop the manifestation of the symptoms so eventually the symptoms return further perpetuating the fallacy that the condition you may have been diagnosed with is "incurable." Notably, natural medicines may also be used in acute situations to stop symptoms without addressing the root cause, also. However, they tend to cause fewer unwanted side effects and work with the body. Thus, it's important to work with medical practitioners who believe healing is possible and who take further steps to help you obtain it.

There have also been numerous patient accounts about encounters with medical professionals who were inconsiderate or abrasive based on how they informed and treated the patient. These types of interactions can scar people and never facilitate healing. Unfortunately, many health professionals may not understand how critical the interactions with patients can be, especially when new diagnoses are given. Essentially, there may be circumstances that have altered your perspective blocking healing.

The name of the condition you were told you have also may be a barrier. We have both mental and emotional responses to the names of diseases with which we or a loved one may be diagnosed. What do you feel when you think of cancer, diabetes, heart disease, high cholesterol, high blood pressure, lupus, hepatitis, HIV, herpes, shingles, infertility, osteoarthritis, rheumatoid arthritis, stroke, kidney disease, lung disease, COPD, asthma, Alzheimer's, dementia, glaucoma, psoriasis, acne, urinary incontinence, anemia, diverticulitis, depression, anxiety, or insomnia? There may be a sense of shame, disgust, or embarrassment. If a loved one died prematurely as a result of one of these conditions, you may feel angry or bitter. Alternatively, you may feel a sense of relief if the "label" of a diagnosis hasn't been pinned on you. Regardless, an initial step toward healing involves releasing the negative mental and emotional associations you have with the diagnosis and recognize you are not your diagnosis. It, whatever it is, doesn't define who you are or make you any less worthy of love and acceptance. So, if you've been sulking about a diagnosis or talking excessively about the disease, then that negative talk can impede healing. You must change your perspective, focus, and conversation.

Another reason healing may not have manifested in your life yet may be due to fear. This fear is rooted in and opposed to faith that is required in order to activate the power of God in our lives for healing or anything else for that matter. God's Word says, "So do not fear, for I am with you; do not be dismayed, for I am your God. I will strengthen you and help you; I will uphold you with my righteous hand."[179] When God looks at us, He doesn't see our blemishes or spots. He only sees our hearts and loves us unconditionally. It pleases Him when we look to our Father in faith with our hearts humbled and yielded because like any good parent, He is eager to bless us and come through on His Word.

Healing's Hide-out

Jesus already paid the price for you to be free from the bondage of sin and death through his suffering, death, and resurrection. When you accepted Him to come live in your heart, everything necessary for a victorious life instantly became available for you—including healing. Thus, healing is *in* you. You only need to understand how to activate your faith to tap into the supernatural power that's already available to heal Christians. You activate this power by meditating on, trusting in, relying on and declaring God's Word with your mouth. Find scriptures on healing and say them to yourself aloud regularly. In order to activate the power in the Word of God, you must only believe what God says about you. Don't waiver, doubt, or fear. Fear is diametrically opposed to faith and quenches the power of God from having access to release blessings. The only way you can effectively do this is by declaring God's Word over you—all of you, spirit, soul and body—on a regular basis.

With time, you will begin to look to God to be your solution and source of healing. You will no longer strive in your own efforts to heal yourself, but you will become completely dependent on Him and His Word, which is what He longed for from the beginning.

Again, no matter what the diagnosis is called and regardless of the pathological mechanisms by which the diseased state manifests in the body, *God's grace covers it all.* Just do your part and allow the Holy Spirit, Who is all knowing, to lead you so healing will be a reality in your life.

During naturopathic medical school, it was appropriately acknowledged that the spiritual aspect of man trumps everything. So be it unto you according to your faith.[180] Trump your flesh. Infuriate the enemy who's kept your mind in bondage for so long regarding your health and put a stop to the schemes. Just say no to Satan's lies and yes to Jesus' blood. It's covered everything, even multiple diagnoses in the same person!

How to be Healed

Being healed isn't supposed to be difficult. There is not a special formula or series of tasks that you must complete in order to qualify for healing as a Christian. You also don't have to have the best health insurance plan or know the right people to get you in to see the best doctors. In fact, the Great Physician is available and ready to see you … and there's no long waiting list or expensive monthly premium! God wants us to be healed, healthy, and pain free. This isn't limited to physical ailments either. God wants us to be emotionally and mentally healthy as well. So again, no matter what diagnosis you were told you "have," you actually have access to the power of the Holy Spirit to release you from all diseases and afflictions.

Accepting healing is similar to accepting salvation. Simply confessing that Jesus is Lord and believing He was raised from the dead is sufficient for salvation.[181] In order to be saved, you had to be aware that you needed to be saved and then informed about how to accept the gift of salvation. Similarly, in order to be healed, you must believe that when Jesus endured crucifixion, the blood that He shed grants us access to God since He was the perfect sacrificial lamb. We were reconciled to God through Jesus. Because of the atonement, we can live the way God originally wanted us to from the beginning of time—free from sin, sickness, and disease. Thus, if you believe in the blood of Jesus, you can *accept* the gift of healing that is readily available for everyone who is part of the body of Christ.

The final step to be healed is that you must confess through your words and actions that you are healed and voila! You *are* healed! This final step is a barrier that prevents many Christians from actually experiencing healing, especially since the amount of time necessary for healing to manifest is variable. The manifestation of healing may not be immediate in your body, but once you believe it, declare it and abide in faith. You are healed. This doesn't mean you are denying that symptoms are present. You are simply declaring God's Words over the situation versus condemning yourself based on what you see because that's not faith. "Faith is the assurance (the confirmation, the title deed) of the things [we] hope for, being the proof of things [we] do not see *and* the conviction of their reality [faith perceiving as real fact what is not revealed to the senses]."[182]

When you receive salvation you also receive God's divine healing. However, because we live in a society where sickness and disease are commonly accepted as the norm, you may need to renew your mind based on what God's Word says about healing. One way to do this is to repetitively train your mind to believe in divine healing by continually confessing aloud that you are healed regardless of your circumstances.

Many of us are unaware of the access we have to God's power. Did you know that God said His Words will not return to Him void?[183] This means all of the promises written in the Bible must be true for anyone who believes in Jesus. God dispatches angels (sometimes on double overtime) to ensure everything recorded in His Word is truth. For example, the Bible says you've been given the power to tread over "all the power of the enemy and nothing by any means shall hurt you." So, if the enemy sends a challenge, threat, or "fiery dart" in your direction, you can say God's Word in that moment and enlist a spiritual army, an angelic legion, to set things right and in alignment with God's Word. Here's a practical example of this. As you take great care of your loaned temple for God, suppose there is an angry driver on the street during your morning jog. Although there is clearly a traffic light where pedestrians have the right-of-way to cross, the impatient, angry driver appears as if he won't stop. The second you see the potential threat, you remember this scripture and pray out loud with authority, "God thank you for giving me power over the enemy, and I know, trust, and believe that nothing by any means shall hurt me." Looking at this situation from many perspectives, there are a number of things that could happen so that you are not harmed. Please consider the following outcomes: 1) The car suddenly malfunctions or gets a flat tire and stops before hitting you. 2) The driver is convicted in his heart and jams on the breaks so you sprint pass confidently. 3) Another vehicle jams into the car before it gets to the intersection. 4) You feel a strong prompting in your spirit to wait so the car passes without harming you. An alternative to these scenarios is that you may not have even been aware of the car, but since you stopped to pick up a toy a kid dropped or since you passionately kissed your spouse before leaving your home, the five-second delay kept you out of harm's way. Finally, even if you do get hit and killed, as a believer, you're going to Heaven when God deems it most appropriate and the transition won't hurt! You'll just suddenly be aware and part of the spiritual realm.

As it relates to health, the same spiritual principles can work! Suppose you notice pain and stiffness in some of the joints of your hands. After you go to see a medical doctor, she diagnoses you with arthritis and writes you a prescription. You thank her and leave. While driving home from the medical center, you turn off the radio and silence your cell phone and begin praying. Then, you start declaring healing scriptures over yourself out loud: "God I thank You for restoring health to me and healing all of my wounds.[184] By the stripes of Jesus I am healed![175] No weapon formed against me shall prosper."[185] As you continue declaring God's Word over the situation, in the spiritual realm, things start shifting. You may not be able to observe any immediate changes with your natural eyes, but your faith and dependence on God to fulfill His promises begins causing shifts, because everything we sense in the physical realm initially starts in the spiritual realm. In your heart and mind, you do not believe or dwell on the diagnosis. Instead, you believe, accept, and hope for an expeditious, full recovery. Regardless of whether you get the prescription and take it (in some cases it may be prudent), you *know* God will come through on His Word, and you are healed. The manifestation of the healing may take a while for you and others to observe. However, since you think and know in your heart God's Word works, it's already done. You continue living joyfully, undaunted by the diagnosis. You also continue speaking scriptures over yourself out loud, especially if symptoms come. You open your heart to hear what the Holy Spirit wants you to do regarding the matter and you obey.

Regardless of the details of the situation, God's Word will become truth in every circumstance when we believe it and hold on to it in faith *knowing* it is truth—no doubt, no fear, only faith. The Word is always available for believers to live with power and authority. We only need to open our mouths and declare God's Word over every area of our lives, particularly our health. Since "the Spirit of Him Who raised up Jesus from the dead dwells in you, [then] He Who raised up Christ *Jesus* from the dead will also restore to life your mortal (short-lived, perishable) bodies through His Spirit Who dwells in you."[186] It's easy for the Holy Spirit to do this! We only have to have faith and *total* reliance on God to bring it to past.

Faith, Fear & Forgiveness

Faith vs. Fear

During Jesus' ministry, He often pointed out when someone's faith was small regarding a matter. He'd say quite pointedly, "Oh ye of little faith."[187] Although He *knew* that God could move in every situation, He consistently observed that others needed to learn how to have faith in God. In the same way, we need to learn to have faith in God for healing. The Bible says "without faith it is impossible to please God."[188] Thus, we must recognize the importance of abiding in faith. What does that mean? Since "faith is the substance of things hoped for, the evidence of things not seen,"[189] it means we must persistently be hopeful and know that what we are hoping for is coming even though we can't see it yet. Since God isn't a respecter of persons, He will do the same for you as He's done for others in the past.[190,191] The key is to operate in faith. Studying biblical accounts of how people were delivered from illness and disease in the Old and New testaments can increase your faith. Here are a few examples for further study and meditation:

- Hannah and infertility (1 Samuel 2:21)
- Elisha and the dead child (2 Kings 4:8-37)
- The man possessed by demons (Mark 5:1-20)

- The woman with the issue of blood (Luke 8:43-48)
- Lazarus raised from the dead (John 11:38-44)

Fear contrasts faith. Jesus was also very clear in His directives about what we should do with fear of illness and disease. Jesus had no fear and reminded others to do the same by saying things like, "Do not be afraid. Just have faith."[192] Fear is essentially the opposite of faith, and it's impossible to operate in faith and fear simultaneously regarding a certain matter. For this reason, as it relates to healing, you can't be fearful about an illness or diagnosis or its effects on your physical body. Remember, you are technically a spirit living in the body. Your spirit is capable of being more powerful than the body it lives in. However, the body must be trained to live in subjection to your spirit, which is intimately connected to the Holy Spirit. The body can be trained by the following:

- Meditating on the Word of God
- Listening to messages by teachers and preachers who are filled with the Holy Spirit
- Praying (both with your understanding and in the Spirit)
- Fasting

Be mindful that there are *good* types of fear that shouldn't be confused with the type of fear that's generally associated with sickness and disease. The fear associated with sickness and disease "brings with it the thought of punishment."[193] However, if you have a sense that your safety may be compromised, this is an indication of another type of fear and you need to use this cue as an indication to move to a safer place. This "alarm" type of fear helps us establish boundaries for ourselves that protect us. There is also a reverential fear of the Lord. This type of fear "is the beginning of all wisdom"[194] because if we persistently recognized the sovereignty of God and feared Him out of reverence, we would not want to or desire to sin. This type of fear is wise. Reverential fear is also protective in nature, because just as parents set limitations for the safety of their children, God does the same with us by setting the standard throughout His Word and guiding us daily through the Holy Spirit at work in us. Thus, reverentially "fearing" Him can keep us out of trouble.

Forgiveness

Sometimes healing can come through forgiveness. "Forgiveness and releasing anyone who has offended us is of monumental importance. This is the road to freedom and good health."[195] When we hold on to negative thoughts and memories from the past, it provides an opportunity for the enemy to divert our attention away from what God has already promised us. For this reason, it's important that we let go of past grievances and move forward optimistically following promptings by the Holy Spirit. The first book of Peter says to "(cast) the whole of your care [all your anxieties, all your worries, all your concerns, once and for all] on Him, for He cares for you affectionately *and* cares about you watchfully."[196] This means that God doesn't want us in a state of anxiety or worry, because ultimately, it will be bad for our health in multifaceted ways: spiritually, mentally and physically.

How to Forgive

Forgiveness is a decision. In order to forgive effectively you must willingly choose to let go of any hurt caused by an individual, a group of people, or a circumstance. Thus, in order for it to happen, in your mind, you must make a choice not to hold others responsible for what they've done in the past. Ask the Holy Spirit to teach you how clear the slate of the offender(s) in your heart and mind regardless of the depth of pain you experienced. If you need to forgive others, aim to clear them of the offense so you perceive them as you did originally before any issues arose. Receive them in a loving manner just as Christ loves and accepts us regardless of our pasts. Of course, this doesn't mean you should allow people to disregard personal boundaries that threaten your safety. If safety is an issue, you should still forgive the person but ensure safety precautions are taken so the person no longer has an opportunity to hurt you. Then, as a child of God, reflect His character through forgiveness. It can expedite your healing and be a testament regarding just how great and awesome God's love is. You could be a light in the situation bringing God glory.

There are also practical ways to make forgiveness tangible. Various options include contacting the person to have a conversation during which you tell them you've forgiven them (regardless of whether they've expressed remorse), write a letter to them (that may or may not be delivered) releasing them of the offense, imagine having a conversation with the person, visit their grave site, etc. Whatever you need to do—regardless of where or when it happens—forgive. Forgiveness on some level is *always* part of the healing process.

Forgiving Yourself

Interestingly, you may not need to forgive another person. You may need to forgive yourself for making a decision or some choices that have led to repercussions you still may be dealing with now. If this is the case, "cut yourself some slack." Accept the reality that no one is perfect. One of the best ways to determine if you need to forgive yourself is to do a complete self-assessment to pinpoint whether you *really* love yourself for who you are including your imperfections. This may be a challenging task for you. One practical way to accomplish this is to talk to a close friend or journal about any areas of your life where there is lingering regret. Then notice if you have any negative emotions towards yourself while reflecting on the situation. If so, you probably need to forgive yourself. However, in order to completely relinquish all grudges and bitterness, you must determine what's left. What traces of your past still negatively impact your present and future? Are there actions you can take to let it go? The Holy Spirit is excellent at revealing these things to us if we are willing to be honest with ourselves. Do you love and accept yourself completely? If not, forgiveness is necessary.

You can use the same practical strategies of forgiving other people in order to forgive yourself. However, simply forgive the person you were at the time you made the "life changing" decision. For example, perhaps you made some poor choices regarding the character of people you've dated in the past. If so, forgive yourself for getting involved with that particular person or people. One pastor very succinctly stated, "The choice that we make for a person to date, court, become engaged to or marry...any time we make such a choice, we are reflecting our spiritual level at the time we make it."[197] Since spiritual growth takes time, we really should forgive ourselves for making poor decisions when we didn't know or understand how to live according to the Spirit. Alternatively, you may have made a bad decision regarding employment or being business partners with someone. Again, filtering choices like this through the Holy Spirit, can help us make better, wiser decisions.

Finally, be mindful that we are required to forgive. Mark 11:26 says, "But if you do not forgive, neither will your Father in heaven forgive your failings and shortcomings." Honestly, if you simply forgive for this reason alone, it will be well worth letting go of the past. No one is worth you not being in good standing with God. We have all sinned and will likely continue to mess up periodically. Because of this, we need to know beyond all reasonable doubt that when we mess up we will be forgiven. So press onward toward the mark of the higher calling and embrace forgiveness just as God forgives us.

God-reliant vs. Self-reliant: Hidden Healing Impediments

Sometimes your healing may be impeded by self-effort. When you become the "expert" at addressing the diagnosis there's no leeway for God to get glory from the situation. Over time and with deceptive success, you may subconsciously perceive yourself as a "god" over the situation. Unfortunately, your expertise has caused another condition, or sequelae, that God loathes—pride. "God opposes the proud, but shows favor to the humble."[198]

Job's account in the Old Testament is reflective of how God feels when we become prideful and attempt to control things by our own power and self-effort. Most of the book of Job includes long diatribes from Job and a few ineffectual responses from his friends. Then, in Chapter 33 a young associate named Elihu addresses the core issue by asking Job "Why do you contend against (God)? For He does not give account of any of His actions. [Sufficient for us it should be to know that it is He who does them.]" In other words, Elihu was essentially "calling Job out" because of Job's self-perceived righteousness and integrity. Meanwhile, God was not pleased though because Job had been "blameless and upright." Numerous tragic events altered Job's perspective because his livestock and camels were stolen, his sheep were burned, all of his kids were killed in a tornado, and he was stricken with disfiguring painful sores. As a result, Job questioned God and began to feel as if he was being treated unfairly since he had lived upright. Slowly, Job became prideful and God responded rather succinctly about how He felt regarding the matter of Job's heart:

> 7 Gird up your loins now like a man; I will demand of you, and you answer Me.
> 8 Will you also annul (set aside and render void) My judgment? Will you condemn Me [your God], that you may [appear] righteous *and* justified?
> 9 Have you an arm like God? Or can you thunder with a voice like His?
> 10 [Since you question the manner of the Almighty's rule] deck yourself now with the excellency *and* dignity [of the Supreme Ruler, and yourself undertake the government of the world

if you are so wise], *and* array yourself with honor and majesty.

11 Pour forth the overflowings of your anger, and look on everyone who is proud and abase him;

12 Look on everyone who is proud and bring him low, and tread down the wicked where they stand [if you are so able, Job].

13 [Bury and] hide them all in the dust together; [and] shut them up [in the prison house of death].

14 [If you can do all this, Job, proving yourself of divine might] then will I [God] praise you also [and acknowledge that] your own right hand can save you.

God made it very clear that He is sovereign and Job needed to recognize His authority. Fortunately, Job repented and the Lord gave Job twice as much as he had before.[199]

In lieu of your situation, perhaps there is a hint of pride or maybe a whole bucket of it that's hindering the flow of the anointing where healing is readily available. If so, the best way to address it is the same way Job did. Admit you are trying to heal yourself through self-effort and recognize that God is sovereign over everything. Admit and acknowledge that you need His help. Once you have repented, ask the Holy Spirit to guide you to truth regarding the situation so you can be healed.

Centenarians and God's Sovereignty

The simplicity of the stories of many people who've lived to be 100 years or more continues to baffle the medical community.

Despite one's efforts at eating a "(healthy) diet, exercising, not smoking, keeping weight under control and (limiting) alcohol consumption," there really are no concrete rules dictating how one can *truly* be healthy or at least when "healthy" is associated with longevity.[200] One study tracked and assessed the lifestyles and habits of centenarians and super centenarians (age 110 and older). "Nearly 40% are overweight (with 8% obese), just under 45% describe only moderate exercise (20% never exercising at all), and nearly 40% are smokers (averaging 31 years)... No depression or other psychiatric illnesses were issues and collectively the group had 60% lower rates of heart disease, high blood pressure, and stroke than on average." The referenced study further noted the only common theme associated with the centenarians' longevity was that they did not hold on to stress and generally had positive outlooks about life, which are definitely options for believers!

Ultimately, the power we have to walk in divine health rests in the grace of God that is available for all believers who receive it. "After doing all the healthy (things) everyone tells you to do, you've got to recognize that it's not divine health if God is not the source of your health."[201] The point here is not to imply that eating vegetables isn't really that important. However, this is simply an admission that God is sovereign. If He extends an abundance of grace as you continue making regular trips to fast food restaurants or habitually getting the "not-so-healthy" options when grocery shopping, so be it. He's God. Just remember, "do not be wise in your own eyes; fear the Lord and turn away from evil. It will be healing to your body and refreshment to your bones."[202]

Prayer, Confession and Healing

As Christians, we possess a uniquely empowering form of communication with the Creator of the universe—prayer. Interestingly, God will not do anything on the Earth until one of us requests it through prayer. As a result, we play an integral role in things occurring here on earth in accordance with God's will. Why is praying so challenging? It may seem challenging if prayer is approached as a ritualistic task that must be done daily. With this approach, there's no focus on your relationship or intimacy with God. Prayer should be more like free flowing conversation instead of a task. Another potential challenge may be due to unfounded religious quotas that a certain amount of time in prayer is required in order for prayers to be answered. Another glitch in one's prayer life could be rooted in rituals. Are you consistently praying the same thing the same way? Monotony in many arenas can lead to boredom. Thus, it's also important to recognize both the necessity of spontaneity in prayer as well as how faith building it can be. Once you begin seeing results, it gets *really* fun and you will look forward to it!

Similarly to setting a lunch date with a friend, we should set aside specific time to pray and interact with God. It's a good time to open your heart and share how much you love and appreciate God for everything He is and the great things He's done and will eventually do during the most appropriate season. If you have other concerns, you can openly and freely share everything on your heart and in your mind without fear of judgment or loss of love. He loves you completely, no matter what.

As it relates to healing, you can pray about your health and the health of your family and friends. Praying once is sufficient, though prayer "addendums" are fine as you become more aware of any other obstacles. We are instructed in Matthew 7:7 to "Ask and it will be given to you; seek and you will find; knock and the door will be opened to you." Once you've asked for healing, you can repetitively thank God for answering your prayer. We should be diligent and faithful in our expectation of a life that's saturated, "exceeding abundantly," with God's grace. Just persistently abide in faith, believe you are already healed and praise and thank God for healing you!

It's possible that some of you may feel discouraged because you feel like you've been doing these things for years, yet you're still not healed. If this is the case, perhaps it's not your persistence in prayer that needs to change, but *what* you are praying. Remember since "God's word will not return to Him void,"[183]—meaning it must come to pass—pray God's Word. Literally, find scriptures based on what you are believing for to help increase your faith. You are God's child. He takes care of His children. The promises in His Word are intended for your benefit. Be wise and use them.

It's also important to recognize that "faith comes by hearing and hearing by the word of God." Thus, something must be said aloud in order for faith to increase. Apostle John Eckhardt had an awesome revelation regarding praying God's word aloud and has compiled several books with prayer confessions, many of which are scripturally based. This makes it super easy to incorporate declaring God's Word in your life during your prayer time with God. He clarifies the importance of saying the prayers aloud based on the following:

Confessing the word of God is an important part of every believer's spiritual life. Christianity is called *the great confession.* Salvation comes from confessing with the mouth. The mouth is connected to the heart. The word of God released from your mouth will be planted in your heart. Faith is released from the mouth. The mouth can only release what is in the heart. Faith in the heart that is released through the mouth can move mountains.

There also may be barriers to breakthrough in the area healing if you've not received your heavenly prayer language or if you don't use it regularly. Praying in the Spirit releases even greater power because you unconsciously pray the perfect will of God.[203] Yielding your tongue to the Holy Spirit can address aspects of healing that you don't fully understand or know to pray. A good example of this is would be apparent from the prayer of a physician yielded to the Great Physician. If the doctor was diagnosed with hypertension, he could pray, "Dear God, I plead the blood of Jesus over every blood vessel in my body. I bind any inflammatory activity that would negatively affect the endothelial cells lining my blood vessels and heart anywhere within my cardiovascular system attempting to promote atherosclerotic plaque formation. I plead the blood of Jesus over my nervous system and kidneys and command that the power of God be released in my body to regulate a proper baroreceptor response as well as balanced hormonal regulation of my renin-angiotensin-aldosterone system so my blood pressure is not high. I have the mind of Christ and am not anxious regarding this matter so there is no sympathetic dominance in my nervous system any longer." Many people not formally trained in pathology wouldn't know specifically what to say. Therefore, you'd have an advantage of asking God to do things you don't know or understand by praying in the Spirit. Additionally, since our current understanding about how the body works continues to expand, what a formally trained doctor prays today will also seem insufficient compared to a doctor's prayer in the future. Praying in the Spirit works for healing as well as other aspects of our lives. Tap into a higher level of power and seek out ministries that teach parishioners who understand the benefits to pray in the Spirit.

We also must be aware of how our prayers are dependent on our confession. We shouldn't pray for healing and deliverance then confess later on or even think in our minds, "Well, I guess it's just not God's will for me to be healed." God *wants* us to live in the full manifestation of glory that He originally intended since the beginning of time. However, it's our responsibility not to curse the promises we are entitled to as children of God regardless of how long it takes for healing to manifest. One savvy minister said that every time we speak, our words are like seeds that will eventually produce fruit that's either positive or negative. Thus, if we attend to the things we say, our experiences in life can change for the better. Remember that "death and life are in the power of the tongue, and they who indulge in it shall eat the fruit of it [for death or life]."[204]

What we say has a lot of power, and our words can change situations for better or worse. "In speaking the word of God, you release into your life the electrifying power that raised Jesus from the grave."[205] Angels are released on assignments based on our prayers. According to Hebrews 4:14-16, we should trust our connection to God through Jesus based on the following:

> **14** Inasmuch then as we have a great High Priest Who has [already] ascended *and* passed through the heavens, Jesus the Son of God, let us hold fast our confession [of faith in Him].
>
> **15** For we do not have a High Priest Who is unable to understand *and* sympathize *and* have a shared feeling with our weaknesses *and* infirmities *and* liability to the assaults of temptation, but One Who has been tempted in every respect as we are, yet without sinning.
>
> **16** Let us then fearlessly *and* confidently *and* boldly draw near to the throne of grace (the throne of God's unmerited favor to us sinners), that we may receive mercy [for our failures] and find grace to help in good time for every need [appropriate help and well-timed help, coming just when we need it].

According to this passage, Jesus already overcame sin of every type and paid the price for it as the perfect sacrifice. Through His blood, we can receive God's grace and mercy. So, if we are ever in need of *anything*—healing, financial breakthrough, mending of broken relationships, career guidance—God is faithful. We can boldly ask for help and trust that our prayers will be answered in the right way at the right time. Matthew 21:22 says, "If you believe, you will receive whatever you ask for in prayer." This means once we finish praying, we need to believe in faith that it's done. This includes following up our prayers with actions that support we believe that our prayers will be answered. So start taking inventory of your words both in prayer and conversation in order to activate the power of God in your life for healing as well as other areas too!

Aside from prayer, confession of the Word and fasting, there are several other ways to be healed as outlined in John Eckhardt's book *Prayers that Bring Healing.* If you are expecting to be healed, be aware of these potential avenues for God to release His miraculous healing power in your life:

- Healing through faith: This is intimately tied to confession, but is anchored in your heart truly believing that you are healed. Though faith, you persistently, actively, repetitively cast down thoughts antagonistic to the promises of God regarding healing and focus on what God said, not the doctor.
- Healing through the presence of God, virtue and touch: (Mark 5:29-30) Just as the lady with uncontrolled bleeding touched a fringe on Jesus' garment and was

healed, the same virtue is available in pure worship. Simply reach up and touch Him.

- Healing through the laying on of hands: When God's anointing is available for believers, healing may come through a willing vessel—either a minister or another believer obeying the Holy Spirit. Charged with the power of God, when this person touches someone with illness or disease, the ailment departs.

- Healing through deliverance: Sometimes sickness is blatantly associated with a demonic spirit. In these cases, the impediment leaves once the person has been delivered from the demonic spirit.

- Healing through breaking curses: This is often useful for genetically related conditions that tend to "run in families." We have authority to inform the devil by declaration of the curse being broken, that generational curses don't have our permission to remain in our bodies.

- Healing through anointing oil: Symbolically, anointing oil represents the Holy Spirit, which drives out illnesses and infirmities by breaking yokes of bondage.

- Healing through the gifts of healing: God has endowed us with various gifts like healing. We have been empowered to do even greater works than Jesus. (John 14:12 and 1 Corinthians 12:9)

- Healing through cloths: Just as people were healed from pieces of cloth that Paul touched, (Acts 19:11-12) the same is still possible today.

An additional consideration for healing is as follows:

- Healing through holy communion: We are instructed to examine our hearts before taking communion. When we do so, we either open ourselves to healing or damnation. (1 Corinthians 11:28-30)

Always remember that with God all things are possible! He extends His love and grace so we can be healed in a variety of ways not based on anything we do or because we deserve it. We are healed simply because of His goodness. Ultimately, we must keep our faith in Him, not on what we've done or not.

<u>The Body of Christ: Health Harvest Time!</u>
There's a need for the body of Christ to recognize our interconnection as outlined in 1 Corinthians 12:25-26:

> The way God designed our bodies is a model for understanding our lives together as a church: every part dependent on every other part, the parts we mention, the parts we don't, the parts we see and the parts we don't. If one part hurts, every other part is involved in the hurt, and in the healing. If one part flourishes, every other part enters into the exuberance.

When one of us is unhealthy and not fulfilling our purpose, it impacts and affects the entire body of Christ. We are all part of the body of Christ, and we are dependent on one another. It's not a coincidence that this was the analogy used to describe us since God designed the parts of the body to function and work beautifully together in symphony. Although modern medicine divides the body up based on organ systems, that's not how the body actually works! It wasn't designed that way. God doesn't want parts of the body of Christ functioning independently. We need each other. Our health and vitality as individuals is dependent on the health and vitality of all of the members. We can do some awesome things for the kingdom of God together, healthy, and whole!

So, here's the challenge, do your best to care for the vessel God entrusted to you and seek opportunities to share what you learn with others as well. Science supports the positive health benefits associated with kind touch and healthy relationships. So let's start focusing on what matters. Your health individually, our health collectively, and God's will being done on earth depends on our awareness of the issues addressed in this book. Let's make decisions individually that will eventually benefit us collectively. It's all for the glory of God!

~

Beloved, I wish above all things that thou mayest prosper and be in health, even as thy soul prospereth. 3 John 1:2 KJV

Appendix

Fasting, Wellness, and Prayer Centers

Fasting Retreat Center:
True North Fasting Center (Santa Rosa, CA)
- http://www.healthpromoting.com

Wellness Retreat Center:
Wildwood Lifestyle Center & Hospital (Wildwood, GA)
- http://www.wildwoodhealth.org

Prayer Retreat Center:
 House of Prayer International (Hampton, GA)
- http://www.prayersretreat.com

Acknowledgements

To Daddy and Mama, cheers to rabbit food! Thank you for loving and supporting me in my endeavors to make a difference in the world. Thanks for taking me to church and letting me discover and embrace my purpose.

To Angela, thank you for encouraging me to go after my passion and for sharing your signature seasoning strategies with me!

To Aretha, thank you for believing in me and seeing the greatness God put in me when it appeared as if I'd settled.

Thanks Raquez, my terrific nephew, for keeping in touch with your "busy" auntie.

To my accountability team (Nadia, Isha, PA, and LaToya), I'd like to express sincere gratitude and thanks for supporting me with prayers and encouragement during this project. Thanks to Eunice and Paula for sharing your resources for content.

Lastly, thanks to my "buddy," LA, for being patient and helpful during the book writing process.

Naturopathic Medicine

What exactly is naturopathic medicine?

"Naturopathic medicine is a distinct primary health care profession, emphasizing prevention, treatment, and optimal health through the use of therapeutic methods and substances that encourage individuals' inherent self-healing process. The practice of naturopathic medicine includes modern and traditional, scientific, and empirical methods."

www.naturopathic.org

How are naturopathic doctors different than medical doctors?

Naturopathic doctors differ in their approach to medicine because the ultimate goal is for the patient's health to improve. Oftentimes, this does not include the necessity of prescription drugs unless warranted. Naturopathic doctors can write prescriptions for you if needed in licensed states. Medical practice is based on the following principles:

- **The Healing Power of Nature (Vis Medicatrix Naturae):** For Christians, this means doctors recognize the divine healing that takes place in our bodies since God created us!
- **Identify and Treat the Causes (Tolle Causam):** The naturopathic physician will make an effort during treatment to figure out what started any medical issues instead of simply prescribing medication to lessen symptoms.
- **First Do No Harm (Primum Non Nocere):** Naturopathic physicians use a variety of methods to treat patients safely implementing alternative approaches like botanical treatments, pharmaceutical grade supplements, water treatments,

homeopathy, acupuncture, etc.

- **Doctor as Teacher (Docere)**: Naturopathic physicians teach and empower patients to play an active role in the patient's health outcomes.

- **Treat the Whole Person**: Naturopathic physicians take into consideration multiple variables that affect health and consider things like individual physical, mental, spiritual, emotional, genetic, environmental, and social factors.
- **Prevention**: Naturopathic physicians recognize the importance of prevention of disease and proactively assess risk factors for diseases instead of "waiting and watching."

Find a Naturopathic Doctor & Be an Advocate for Change!
If you are interested in receiving medical care from a licensed primary care physician formally trained in naturopathic medicine, you can find one near you by visiting, http://www.naturopathic.org. Once on the site, click on the "Find a Doctor" link and follow the instructions.

Currently, NDs are licensed in the following states:

Alaska	Minnesota
Arizona	Montana
California	New Hampshire
Colorado	North Dakota
Connecticut	Oregon
District of Columbia	Utah
Hawaii	Vermont
Kansas	Washington
Maine	Puerto Rico & the Virgin Islands
Maryland	

If you'd like for naturopathic doctors to be available and accessible in your state, tell your elected officials—senators and representatives—repeatedly. Also, choose health insurance plans that cover services from naturopathic doctors or call your current health insurance company to request that naturopathic doctors be included as providers.

References by Chapter

Chapter 1
[1] Matthew 4:7 AMP
[2] Psalm 32:8-9 AMP

Chapter 2
[3] Helmenstine, A. (n.d). Chemistry of Autumn Leaf Color: How Fall Colors Work. Retrieved September 23, 2014, from http://chemistry.about.com/library/weekly/aa082602a.htm
[4] Hoyert, D.L., Xu, J. (2012). Deaths: Preliminary data for 2011. *National Vital Statistics Reports*, 61(6). Retrieved November 12, 2013 from http://www.cdc.gov/nchs/data/nvsr/nvsr61/nvsr61_06.pdf
[5] John 10:10 AMP
[6] I Peter 5:8 AMP
[7] Mark 4:19 KJV
[8] Philippians 4:13 NKJV
[9] I Peter 2:11 AMP
[10] Romans 12:2 NIV
[11] I John 2:15-16 KJV
[12] Luke 16:13 KJV
[13] Matthew 6:24 KJV
[14] Isaiah 55:11KJV
[15] Acts 1:8 AMP
[16] Acts 2:4 AMP
[17] Ephesians 6:18 AMP
[18] Ephesians 6:16 AMP

Chapter 3
[19] Psalm 139:14 NLT
[20] Psalm 139:13 NIV
[21] Davis-Sivasothy, A. (2011). *The science of black hair: A comprehensive guide to textured hair care*. Stafford, TX: Saja Publishing Company, LLC.
[22] Champe, P. C., Harvey, R. A. , and Ferrier, D. R. (2008). *Lippincott's Illustrated Reviews: Biochemistry, 4th Ed*. Baltimore, MD: Lippincott Williams & Wilkins

23 Jeukendrup, A. & Gleeson, M. (2010). *Sport Nutrition: An Introduction to energy production and performance, 2nd Ed.* Champaign, IL: Human Kinetics, Inc. Retrieved November 8, 2014, from http://www.humankinetics.com/excerpts/excerpts/normal-ranges-of-body-weight-and-body-fat

24 Jawon Medical (n.d.) Body Composition. Retrieved November 18, 2013, from http://www.jawon.com/reng/res/body-composition.html

25 Berstein, R. (2007). *Diabetes Solution: The Complete Guide to Achieving Normal Blood Sugars.* Little, Brown, and Company: New York, NY.

26 Marz, R. (1999). *Medical Nutrition: 2nd Ed.* Portland, OR: Omni-Press.

27 Schoffro-Cook, M. (2013). 25 Ingredients in McDonald's Chicken McNuggets. Retrieved January 3, 2014, from http://www.care2.com/greenliving/25-ingredients-in-mcdonalds-chicken-mcnuggets.html

28 MacWilliam, L. (2009). Nutrient Depletion of Our Foods. Retrieved January, 11, 2014, from http://www.myhealthyhome.com/wp-content/uploads/2011/02/NutrientDepletionofourFoods.pdf

29 Thomas, D. (2007). The mineral depletion of foods available to us as a nation (1940–2002) — A review of the 6th edition of McCance and Widdowson. *Nutrition and Health, 19,* 21–55.

30 Environmental Working Group. (n.d.). *10 Americans* [Video]. Retrieved and viewed January 11, 2014 from http://www.ewg.org/news/videos/10-americans

31 Webb, G. (2014). Genetically Modified Foods (GMOs) – What's the Big Deal. Retrieved January 3, 2014, from http://charlottesville.legalexaminer.com/uncategorized/genetically-modified-foods-gmos-whats-the-big-deal/

32 Organic Consumers Association. (n.d). Countries & Regions With GE Food/Crop Bans. Retrieved January 11, 2014, from http://www.organicconsumers.org/gefood/countrieswithbans.cfm

33 Proverbs 4:7 NKJV

34 U.S. Food and Drug Administration (n.d.). Trans Fat. Retrieved January 6, 2014, from http://www.fda.gov/Food/ucm292278.htm

35 Mozaffarian, D., Aro, A., and Willett, W. (2009). Health effects of trans-fatty acids: experimental and observational evidence. *European Journal of Clinical Nutrition*, 63, S5–S21.

36 Medicine Net (n.d.) Insulin Resistance. Retrieved January 11, 2014, from http://www.medicinenet.com/insulin_resistance/page3.htm

37 Cooper, F. (2008). Interesterification - The Dangerous Replacement for Trans-fats. Retrieved July 2, 2014, from http://www.naturalnews.com/022759_oil_fat_oils.html

38 Enig, M. (2008). Interesterification. Retrieved July 2, 2014, from http://www.westonaprice.org/health-topics/interesterification/

39 Sundram, K., Karupaiah, T., and Hayes, K. (2007). Stearic acid-rich interesterified fat and trans-rich fat raise the LDL/HDL ratio and plasma glucose relative to palm olein in humans. *Nutrition & Metabolism*, 4, 3.

40 World Cancer Research Fund & the American Institute for Cancer Research (2007). *Food, nutrition, physical activity, and the prevention of cancer: A global perspective*. Washington DC: AICR.

41 Simopoulos, A. (2008). The importance of the omega-6/omega-3 fatty acid ratio in cardiovascular disease and other chronic diseases. *Experimental Biology and Medicine, 233*, 674-688.

42 Blasbalg, T., Hibbeln, J., Ramsden, C., et al. (2011). Changes in consumption of omega-3 and omega-6 fatty acids in the United States during the 20th century. *American Journal of Clinical Nutrition, 93*, 950–62.

43 Realini, C., Duckett, S., Brito, G., et al. (2004). Effect of pasture vs. concentrate feeding with or without antioxidants on carcass characteristics, fatty acid composition, and quality of Uruguayan beef. *Meat Science, 66*, 567–577.

44 U.S. Food and Drug Administration. (2013). Phasing Out Certain Antibiotic Use in Farm Animals. Retrieved November 11, 2014, from

http://www.fda.gov/ForConsumers/ConsumerUpdates/ucm37 8100.htm

[45] Love, D., Davis, M., Bassett, A., et al. (2011). Dose imprecision and resistance: Free-choice medicated feeds in industrial food animal production in the United States. *Environmental Health Perspectives, 119* (3) 279-283.

[46] Herna´ndez-Arteseros, J., Barbosa, J, Compano, R., et al. (2002). Analysis of quinolone residues in edible animal products. [Review on the analysis of quinolone antibacterials]. *Journal of Chromatography-A, 945,* 1-24.

[47] Cogliani, C., Goossens, H., & Greko, C. (2011). Restricting antimicrobial use in food animals: Lessons from Europe banning nonessential antibiotic uses in food animals is intended to reduce pools of resistance genes. *Microbe, 6,* 274-279.

[48] Medical News Today. (2013). FDA to Phase Out Non-therapeutic Use of Antibiotics in Food Animals. Retrieved January 1, 2014, from http://www.medicalnewstoday.com/articles/270010.php

[49] U.S. Food and Drug Administration. (2014). FDA's Strategy on Antimicrobial Resistance: Questions and Answers. Retrieved on January 24, 2014, from http://www.fda.gov/AnimalVeterinary/GuidanceComplianceEn forcement/GuidanceforIndustry/ucm216939.htm

[50] Silverman, E. (2014). FDA Plan for Antibiotics in Food-Producing Livestock is Weak: Senators. Retrieved November 14, 2014, from http://blogs.wsj.com/pharmalot/2014/07/29/fda-plan-for-antiobiotics-in-food-producing-livestock-is-weak-senators/

[51] Gandhi, R. & Snedeker, S. (2003). Consumer Concerns About Hormones in Food. Retrieved November 14, 2014, from http://envirocancer.cornell.edu/factsheet/diet/fs37.hormones.cfm

[52] Bartelt-Hunt, S., Snow, D., Kranz, W., et al. (2012). Effect of growth promotants on the occurrence of endogenous and synthetic steroid hormones on feedlot soils and in runoff from beef cattle feeding operations. *Environmental Science & Technology, 46,* 1352–1360.

53 Aksglaede, L., Juul, A., & Leffers, H. (2006). The sensitivity of the child to sex steroids: Possible impact of exogenous estrogens. *Human Reproduction Update,12,* 341–349.

54 Andersson, A. and Skakkebaek, N. (1999). Exposure to exogenous estrogens in food: Possible impact on human development and health. *European Journal of Endcrinology, 140,*477–485.

55 Parker, H. (2010). A sweet problem: Princeton researchers find that high-fructose corn syrup prompts considerably more weight gain. Retrieved on November 11, 2014, from http://www.princeton.edu/main/news/archive/S26/91/22K07/

56 Schoenfeld, L. (2012). The Biochemistry of High Fructose Corn Syrup. Retrieved on January 25, 2014, from http://www.ancestralizeme.com/the-biochemistry-of-high-fructose-corn-syrup/

57 Ferder, L. & Ferder, M. & Inserra, F. (2010). The role of high-fructose corn syrup in metabolic syndrome and hypertension. *Current Hypertension Reports, 12,* 105–112.

58 White, J. (2009). Misconceptions about high-fructose corn syrup: Is it uniquely responsible for obesity, reactive dicarbonyl compounds, and advanced glycation endproducts. *Journal of Nutrition, 139,* 1219S–1227S.

59 U.S. Food and Drug Administration. (2013). High Fructose Corn Syrup: Questions and Answers. Retrieved from. January 25, 2014 , from http://www.fda.gov/food/ingredientspackaginglabeling/foodadditivesingredients/ucm324856.htm

60 Charles, H., Godfray, J., Beddington, J., et al. (2010). Food Security: The Challenge of Feeding 9 Billion People. [Review of global food demand]. *Science, 327,* 812-818.

61 Harvard School of Public Health. (n.d.). Genetically Modified Foods. Retrieved November 24, 2014, from http://www.chgeharvard.org/topic/genetically-modified-foods

62 Monsanto (n.d.) Biotechnology. Retrieved on March 18, 2014, from

http://www.monsanto.com/products/pages/biotechnology.asp x

63 Domingo, J. and Bordonaba, J. (2011). A literature review on the safety assessment of genetically modified plants. *Environment International, 37*, 734–742.

64 Batista, R. and Oliveira, M. (2009). Facts and fiction of genetically engineered food. *Trends in Biotechnology, 27*(5), 277-286.

65 Azadi, H. and Ho, P. (2010). Genetically modified and organic crops in developing countries: A review of options for food security. *Biotechnology Advances, 28*, 160–168.

66 Gillam, C. (2014). *U.S. GMO crops show mix of benefits, concerns. Retrieved April 2, 2014, from* http://www.reuters.com/article/2014/02/24/usda-gmo-report-idUSL1N0LT16M20140224

67 Committee on the Impact of Biotechnology on Farm-Level Economics and Sustainability. (2010). *The Impact of Genetically Engineered Crops on Farm Sustainability in the United States.* Washington, D.C.: National Academies Press.

68 National Research Council. (2004). *Safety of Genetically Engineered Foods: Approaches to Assessing Unintended Health Effects.* Washington, DC: The National Academies Press.

69Cellini, F., Chesson, A., Colquhoun, I., et al. (2004). Unintended effects and their detection in genetically modified crops. *Food and Chemical Toxicology, 42*, 1089–1125.

70 Sciammacco, S. (2014). 200 Groups Call On Obama To Keep Campaign Pledge: Label GMOs Members of Congress hold press conference urging President to support mandatory labeling. *Retrieved January 26, 2014, from* http://www.ewg.org/release/200-groups-call-obama-keep-campaign-pledge-label-gmos

71 Formuzis, A. (2014). Cheerios New Non-GMO Label Tests Food Industry Claims on Labeling. Retrieved January 26, 2014, from http://www.ewg.org/enviroblog/2014/01/cheerios-new-non-gmo-label-tests-food-industry-claims-labeling

72 Young, C. (2013). 7 Most Common Genetically Modified Foods. Retrieved January 31, 2014, from m.huffpost.com/us/entry/4323937

73 Geib, A. (2012). GMO Alert: Top 10 Genetically Modified Foods to Avoid Eating. Retrieved January 31, 2014, from http://www.naturalnews.com/035734_GMOs_foods_dangers.html

74 Le Curieux-Belfond, O., Vandelac, L., Caron, J., et al. (2009). Factors to consider before production and commercialization of aquatic genetically modified organisms: the case of transgenic salmon. [Review of the impacts of transgenic salmon]. *Environmental Science & Policy 12,*170–189.

75 Goldenberg, S. (2013). Canada Approves Production of GM Salmon eggs on Commercial Scale. Retrieved January 31, 2014, from http://www.theguardian.com/environment/2013/nov/25/canada-genetically-modified-salmon-commercial

76 Lipman, F. (2012). What Do Those Codes On Stickers Of Fruits And Some Veggies Mean? Retrieved April 5, 2014, from http://www.drfranklipman.com/what-do-those-codes-on-stickers-of-fruits-and-some-veggies-mean/

77 Mercola, J. (2011). If You Eat Processed Meats, Are You Risking Your Life? Retrieved February 22, 2014, from http://articles.mercola.com/sites/articles/archive/2011/01/22/if-you-eat-processed-meats-youre-risking-your-life.aspx

78 Tricker, A. & Preussmann, R. (1991). Carcinogenic N-nitrosamines in the diet: occurrence, formation, mechanisms and carcinogenic potential. *Mutation Research, 259,* 277–289.

79 Milkowski, A., Garg, H., Coughlin, J., et al. (2010). Nutritional epidemiology in the context of nitric oxide biology: A risk–benefit evaluation for dietary nitrite and nitrate. [Review of the epidemiological data and discussion of the risk–benefit evaluation of dietary nitrite and nitrate in the context of nitric oxide biology]. *Nitric Oxide, 22* (2010) 110–119.

80 Gilchrist, M., Winyard, P., & Benjamin, N. (2010). Dietary nitrate – Good or bad? [Review of recent evidence for the positive and negative effects of inorganic nitrate in humans]. *Nitric Oxide, 22*

(2010) 104–109.

[81] Mercola, J. (2009). MSG: Is This Silent Killer Lurking in Your Kitchen Cabinets. Retrieved February 22, 2014 from http://articles.mercola.com/sites/articles/archive/2009/04/2 1/msg-is-this-silent-killer-lurking-in-your-kitchen-cabinets.aspx

[82] U.S. Food and Drug Administration. (2012). Questions and Answers on Monosodium glutamate (MSG). Retrieved February 22, 2014, from http://www.fda.gov/food/ingredientspackaginglabeling/fooda dditivesingredients/ucm328728.htm

[83] Choi, D. and Rothman, S. (1990). The role of glutamate neurotoxicity in hypoxic-ischemial neuronal death. *Annual Review of Neuroscience, 13*, 171-82.

[84] Shivasharan, B., Nagakannan, P., Thippeswamy, B., et al. (2013). Protective effect of *calendula officinalis* l. flowers against monosodium glutamate induced oxidative stress and excitotoxic brain damage in rats. *Indian Journal of Clinical Biochemistry, 28*(3), 292–298.

[85] Iverson, F. (1999). In vivo studies on butylated hydroxyanisole, *Food and Chemical Toxicology 37*, 993-997.

[86] Bosch, L. (2010). Top 10 Food Additives to Avoid. Retrieved February 22, 2014, from http://foodmatters.tv/articles-1/top-10-food-additives-to-avoid

[87] Botterweck, A., Verhagen, H., Goldbohm, R., et al. (2000). Intake of butylated hydroxyanisole and butylated hydroxytoluene and stomach cancer risk: Results from analyses in the Netherlands cohort study. *Food and Chemical Toxicology, 38*, 599-605.

[88] Aspinall, R., Saunders, R., Pautsch, W., et. al. (1980). The biological properties of aspartame: Effects on a variety of physiological parameters related to inflammation and metabolism. *Journal of Environmental Pathology & Toxicology, 3*, 387–395.

[89] Castro, R. (2013). Can I Use Artificial Sweeteners if I have Diabetes? Retrieved November 14, 2014, from http://www.mayoclinic.org/diseases-

conditions/diabetes/expert-answers/artificial-sweeteners/faq-20058038

90 Novick, N. (1985). Aspartame-induced granulomatous panniculitis. *Annals of Internal Medicine.102*, 206–207.

91 Expert Consult (n.d.). Definition of Granulomatous Panniculitis. Retrieved June 6, 2014, from http://www.expertconsultbook.com/expertconsult/ob/book.do?method=display&type=bookPage&decorator=none&eid=4-u1.0-B978-0-443-06654-2..00002-0--s0370&isbn=978-0-443-06654-2

92 National Cancer Institute (n.d.). Formaldehyde and Cancer Risks. Retrieved June 7, 2014, from http://www.cancer.gov/cancertopics/factsheet/Risk/formaldehyde

93Susanna, K. (2013).11 Food Ingredients Banned Outside the U.S. That We Eat. Retrieved June 7, 2014, from http://gma.yahoo.com/11-food-ingredients-banned-outside-u-eat-101120572--abc-news-topstories.html

94 Hari, V. (n.d.). Before You Ever Buy Bread Again...Read This! (And Find The Healthiest Bread On The Market). Retrieved June 7, 2014 from http://foodbabe.com/tag/azodicarbonamide/

95 U.S. Food and Drug Administration. (2014). Ingredients Packaging Labeling & Food Additives Ingredients. Retrieved June 7, 2014, from http://www.fda.gov/Food/IngredientsPackagingLabeling/FoodAdditivesIngredients/ucm387497.htm

96 Mendes Da Costa, M., Duarte, A., , Capela-Silva, F., et al. (2012). Liver morphologic changes induced by semicarbazide. *The FASEB Journal, 26*, 478.2.

97 U.S. Food and Drug Administration. (n.d.). Code of Federal Regulations, Title 21 - Food and Drug Administration Department of Health and Human Services. Retrieved February 22, 2014, from http://www.accessdata.fda.gov/scripts/cdrh/cfdocs/cfcfr/cfrsearch.cfm?fr=101.22

98Buczynski, B. (2013). 10+ Scary Reasons To Avoid Artificial Food Coloring. Retrieved May 29, 2014, from http://www.care2.com/greenliving/10-scary-reasons-to-avoid-artificial-food-coloring.html

[99]Rowe, R., Sheskey, P., & Quinn, M. (Eds.). (2009). Handbook of Pharmaceutical Excipients, 6th Edition. Grayslake, IL: Pharmaceutical Press and American Pharmacists Association.

[100] Carrera, A. (2013). Is Red 40 Food Coloring Dangerous to Your Health? Retrieved May 29, 2014, from http://www.livestrong.com/article/445428-is-red-40-food-coloring-dangerous-to-your-health/

[101] Davidson, P., Sofos, J., & Branen, A. (Eds.). (2005). *Antimicrobials in Food, 3rd Edition*. Boca Raton, FL: CRC Press.

[102] U.S. Food and Drug Administration. (n.d.). Code of Federal Regulations, Title 21 - Food and Drug Administration Department of Health and Human Services. Retrieved February 27, 2014, from http://www.accessdata.fda.gov/scripts/cdrh/cfdocs/cfcfr/CFRSearch.cfm?fr=184.1733

[103] McCann, D., Barrett, A., Cooper, A., et. al. (2007). Food additives and hyperactive behaviour in 3-year-old and 8/9-year-old children in the community: A randomised, double-blinded, placebo-controlled trial. *Lancet, 370,* 1560–1567.

[104] Canon, T. (2014). What Is Sprayed On Produce After Harvest? Retrieved June 12, 2014, from http://ethicalfoods.com/sprayed-produce-harvest/

[105] Cox, C. (1997). Fumigant Fact Sheet: Sulfuryl Fluoride. *Journal of Pesticide Reform, 17* (2), 17-20.

[106] Feron, V., Flemming, R., Cassee, J., et.al. (2002). International issues on human health effects of exposure to chemical mixtures. *Environmental Health Perspectives. 110*(6), 893–899.

[107] Jain, S. & Hochstein, P. (1979). Generation of superoxide radicals by hydrazine: Its role in phenylhydrazine-induced hemolytic anemia. *Biochemicha et Biophysica Acta, 586,* 128-136.

[108] Bjørling-Poulsen, M., Andersen, H. & Grandjean P. (2008). Potential developmental neurotoxicity of pesticides used in Europe. *Environmental Health* 2008,7, 50.

[109] United States Environmental Protection Agency Prevention.

(1994). R.E.D. Facts: Maleic Hydrazide, Pesticides And Toxic Substances (EPA-738-F-94-009). Retrieved June 12, 2014 from http://www.epa.gov/oppsrrd1/REDs/factsheets/0381fact.pdf
[110] Zander, A. & Bunning, M. (2010). Guide to Washing Fresh Produce. Retrieved November 24, 2014, from http://www.ext.colostate.edu/pubs/foodnut/09380.pdf
[111] Luke 2:49 KJV

Chapter 4
[112] Kenneth Copeland Ministries. (n.d.). Understanding the Soul. Retrieved November 20, 2013, from http://www.kcm.org/real-help/article/understanding-soul
[113] Wommack, A. (n.d.). Spirit, Soul and Body. Retrieved November 20, 2013, from http://www.awmi.net/extra/article/spirit_soul
[114] Ephesians 4:26 NIV
[115] Matthew 6:33 KJV
[116] Houdmann, M. (n.d.) Is gluttony a sin? What does the Bible say about overeating? Retrieved November 21, 2013, from http://www.gotquestions.org/gluttony-sin.html
[117] Wansink, B. (2006). *Mindless Eating: Why We Eat More Than We Think*. New York, NY: Bantam Dell of Random House, Inc.
[118] Centers for Disease Control. (2013). Exercise or Physical Activity Retrieved November 22, 2013, from http://www.cdc.gov/nchs/fastats/exercise.htm
[119] Bertrand, P. & Bertrand, R. (2010). Serotonin release and uptake in the gastrointestinal tract. *Autonomic Neuroscience: Basic and Clinical, 153*, 47–57.
[120] Firk, C. & Markus, C.R. (2007). Serotonin by stress interaction: A susceptibility factor for the development of depression? *Journal of Psychopharmacology, 21*(5), 538–544.
[121] Cowen, P. (2002). Cortisol, serotonin and depression: all stressed out? *British Journal of Psychiatry, 180*, 99-100.
[122] Chaouloff, F., Berton, O., & Mormède, P. (1999). Serotonin and Stress. *Neuropsychopharmacology, 21*, 28S-32S.

[123] Anderwald, C., Brabant, G., Bernroider, E., et al. (2003). Insulin-dependent modulation of plasma ghrelin and leptin concentrations is less pronounced in type 2 diabetic patients. *Diabetes, 52*, 1792-1798.

[124] Koç, F., Tokaç, M., Kocabaş, V., et al. (2011). Ghrelin, resistin and leptin in metabolic syndrome. *European Journal of General Medicine, 8*(2), 92-7.

[125] Spiegel, K., Tasali, E., Penev, P., et al. (2004). Brief communication: Sleep curtailment in healthy young men is associated with decreased leptin levels, elevated ghrelin levels, and increased hunger and appetite. *Annals of Internal Medicine, 141*(11), 846-850.

[126] Proverbs 27:3a AMP

[127] Terkeurst, L. (2010). *Made to Crave*. Grand Rapids, MI: Zondervan.

[128] Gripshover, S. & Markman, E. (2013). Teaching young children a theory of nutrition: Conceptual change and the potential for increased vegetable consumption. *Psychological Science, 24*: 1541-1553.

[129] Oyserman, D., Fryberg, S., and Yoder, N. (2007). Identity-based motivation and health. *Journal of Personality and Social Psychology, 93*, 1011–1027.

[130] Ephesians 2:19 NIV

[131] Proverbs 4:7 AMP

[132] Lazarony, L. (n.d.). 17 Tips for Buying Organic Food on the Cheap. Retrieved February 28, 2014, from http://www.bankrate.com/brm/news/cheap/20040901a2.asp

[133] Breed, M. (n.d.). 10 Ways to Save Money Buying Fresh Produce – Fruits and Vegetables. Retrieved February 28, 2014, from http://www.moneycrashers.com/how-to-save-money-buying-fruits-and-vegetables/

Chapter 5

[134] I Samuel 16:7b

[135] Beers, M., Porter, R., Jones, T., et al. (Eds.). (2006). *The Merck Manual: 18th Ed.* Whitehouse Station, NJ: Merck Research Laboratories.

[136] Gaby, Alan. *Nutritional Medicine.* Concord, NH: Fritz Perlberg Publishing, 2011

[137] Pines, A., Raafat, H., Lynn, A. et al. (1984). Clinical trial of microcrystalline hydroxyapatite compound ('ossopan') in the prevention of osteoporosis due to corticosteroid therapy. *Current Medical Research and Opinion. 8*(10), 734-742.

[138] Liu, S., Willett, W., Stampfer, M., et al. (2000). A prospective study of dietary glycemic load, carbohydrate intake, and risk of coronary heart disease in US women. *American Journal of Clinical Nutrition, 71,* 1455–1461.

[139] Dolson, L. (2013). How To Read a Nutrition Label. Retrieved March 8, 2014, from http://lowcarbdiets.about.com/od/nutrition/ss/nutritionlabels_6.htm

[140] James 2:17 AMP

[141] Matthew 6:34 AMP

[142] Kiernan, B. (2012). Grass Fed versus Corn Fed: You Are What Your Food Eats. Retrieved March 12, 2012 from http://www.globalaginvesting.com/news/blogdetail?contentid=1479

[143] Mercola, J. (2012). One of the Worst Ways to Eat Eggs. Retrieved March 12, 2014 from http://articles.mercola.com/sites/articles/archive/2012/03/19/caged-vs-free-range-chicken-eggs.aspx

[144] Craig, W. (2009). Health effects of vegan diets. *American Journal of Clinical Nutrition, 89*(suppl), 1627S–1633S.

[145] Theobald, H., Chowienczyk, P., Whittall, R, et al. (2004). LDL cholesterol – raising effect of low-dose docosahexaenoic acid in middle-aged men and women. *American Journal of Clinical Nutrition, 79,* 558-563.

[146] WebMD. (n.d.) Vitamin D Deficiency. Retrieved March 18, 2014, from http://www.webmd.com/food-recipes/vitamin-d-deficiency

[147] Mercola, J. (2012). 26 out of 54 People Who Avoided These Foods Got a Brain-Destroying Vitamin B12 Deficiency. Retrieved March 18, 2014 from http://articles.mercola.com/sites/articles/archive/2012/02/15/how-to-avoid-the-most-dangerous-side-effect-of-veganism.aspx

[148] Mercola, J. (2011). The Cholesterol Myths that may be harming your Health. Retrieved March 28, 2014 from http://articles.mercola.com/sites/articles/archive/2011/10/22/debunking-the-science-behind-lowering-cholesterol-levels.aspx

[149] Kummerow, F. (2013). Two lipids in the diet, rather than cholesterol, are responsible for heart failure and stroke *Clinical Lipidology, 8*(3):289-294.

[150] Kummerow, F. interviewed by Wilson, H. (2013). Correlation between Oxysterol Consumption and Heart Disease. Eat Your Eggs. Retrieved March 28, 2013, from http://preventivecardiologist.wordpress.com/category/atherosclerosis-2/

[151] Kummerow, F., Olinescu, R., Fleischer, L., et al. (2000) The relationship of oxidized lipids to coronary artery stenosis. *Atherosclerosis, 149*, 181–190.

[152] Schoenian, S. (n.d.). The truth about grain: Feeding grain to small ruminants. Retrieved March 29, 2014, from http://www.sheepandgoat.com/articles/graintruth.html

[153] Mercola, J. (2010). Coconut Oil: This Cooking Oil Is a Powerful Virus-Destroyer and Antibiotic. Retrieved March 29, 2014, from http://articles.mercola.com/sites/articles/archive/2010/10/22/coconut-oil-and-saturated-fats-can-make-you-healthy.aspx

[154] Good, J. (2012). Healthiest Cooking Oil Chart with Smoke Points. Retrieved March 29, 2014, from

https://jonbarron.org/article/healthiest-cooking-oil-chart-smoke-points#.UzdGzf25ilw

[155] Kershner, K. (n.d.). How Reverse Osmosis Works. Retrieved April 5, 2014, from http://science.howstuffworks.com/reverse-osmosis3.htm

[156] Wright, C. (2013). Reverse osmosis, distilled, spring or ionized? Experts weigh in on water. Retrieved March 22, 2014, from http://www.naturalnews.com/043289_reverse_osmosis_water_treatment_ph_balance.html

[157] Mercola, J. (n.d.). How Drinking More Spring or Filtered Water Can Improve Every Facet of Your Health. Retrieved March 22, 2014, from http://www.mercola.com/article/water.htm

[158] Marchese, M. (2011). The Truth About Plastic Water Bottles. Retrieved November 14, 2014, from http://www.smart-publications.com/articles/the-truth-about-plastic-water-bottles

[159] Alexander, S. (n.d.). 4 Great Benefits of Seasonal Eating. Retrieved April 5, 2014, from http://eatlocalgrown.com/article/11365-4-great-benefits-of-seasonal-eating.html

[160] Mercola, J. & Droege, R. (2004). How to Find out if You Have Food and Chemical Sensitivities. Retrieved April 5, 2014, from http://articles.mercola.com/sites/articles/archive/2004/04/03/chemical-sensitivities.aspx

[161] Mercola, J. (2013). Japanese Doctor Confirms Benefits of Working Out Less, but More Intensely. Retrieved April 19, 2014, from http://fitness.mercola.com/sites/fitness/archive/2013/04/12/tabata-workout.aspx

[162] Hillman, C., Erickson, K. & Kramer A. (2008). Be smart, exercise your heart: exercise effects on brain and cognition. *Nature Reviews Neuroscience, 9*(1), 58-65.

Chapter 6

[163] Copeland, K. (2009). Fasting and Prayer. Retrieved April 19, 2014, from

http://www.kennethandgloriacopeland.net/57/fasting-and-prayer-by-kenneth-copeland/

[164] Esther Chapters 2-5 KJV

[165] Esther 3:13 NIV

[166] Ester 4:14 NIV

[167] Matthew 4:1-11 KJV

[168] Matthew 6:16-18 AMP

[169] Hagee, J. (1991). *The Power to Heal*. Dallas, Tx: John Hagee & Global Evangelism Television, Inc.

[170] Kail, J. (2013). 4 Spiritual Benefits of Fasting. Retrieved April 19, 2014, from http://www.jakekail.com/4-spiritual-benefits-fasting/

[171] Gregory, S. (n.d.). What is the Daniel Fast? Retrieved November 14, 2014, from http://www.daniel-fast.com/aboutthefast/

[172] Daniel 10:2-3 KJV

[173] All About Fasting. (2008). Intermittent Fasting. Retrieved February 15, 2014, from http://www.allaboutfasting.com/intermittent-fasting.html

[174] Murray, M. & Pizzorno, J. (1998). *Encyclopedia of Natural Medicine: 2nd Ed.* New York: Three Rivers Press.

Chapter 7

[175] Isaiah 53:5 AMP

[176] I Peter 2:24 AMP

[177] Hunter, Joan. (2005). *Healing the Whole Man Handbook*. New Kensington, PA: Whitaker House.

[178] Hagin, Kenneth. (1998). *God's Divine Word on Healing*. Tulsa, OK: Faith Library Publications.

[179] Isaiah 41:10 NIV

[180] Matthew 9:29 AMP

[181] Romans 10:9 AMP

[182] Hebrews 11:1 AMP

[183] Isaiah 55:11 AMP

[184] Jeremiah 30:17 NIV

[185] Isaiah 54:17 NASB

[186] Romans 8:11 AMP

[187] Matthew 8:26 AMP

[188] Hebrews 11:6 NIV
[189] Hebrews 11:1 KJV
[190] Acts 10:34 KJV
[191] Job 34:19 AMP
[192] Luke 8:50 NLT
[193] I John 4:18 AMP
[194] Proverbs 9:10 AMP
[195] McKinney-Hammond, M. (1997). *What to Do Until Love Finds You.* Eugene, OR: Harvest House Publishing.
[196] I Peter 5:7 AMP
[197] Advent Exodus. (2013). The Holy Spirit and Choosing a Mate. [Video]. Retrieved November 14, 2014, from https://www.youtube.com/watch?v=XrqkfZwm8z8
[198] James 4:6 NIV
[199] Job 40:24 AMP
[200] Mercola, J. (2014). How Centenarians Explain Their Longevity. Retrieved April 11, 2014, from http://articles.mercola.com/sites/articles/archive/2014/01/09/centenarians.aspx
[201] Dollar, C. (Minister). (2012). 2012 Ministers' and Leaders' Conference. (Series on Compact Discs – Disc 6, Part 1). College Park, GA: Creflo Dollar Ministries.
[202] Proverbs 3:7-8 NIV
[203] Romans 8:26 AMP
[204] Proverbs 18:21 AMP
[205] Hagee, J. (1991). *The Power to Heal.* Dallas, TX: John Hagee & Global Evangelism Television, Inc.